MADE TO ORDER

The Designing of Animals

MARGARET E. DERRY

MADE TO ORDER

The Designing of Animals

UNIVERSITY OF TORONTO PRESS
Toronto Buffalo London

© University of Toronto Press 2022
Toronto Buffalo London
utorontopress.com

ISBN 978-1-4875-4160-6 (cloth)
ISBN 978-1-4875-4163-7 (EPUB)
ISBN 978-1-4875-4162-0 (PDF)

Library and Archives Canada Cataloguing in Publication

Title: Made to order : the designing of animals / Margaret E. Derry.
Names: Derry, Margaret E. (Margaret Elsinor), 1945– author.
Description: Includes bibliographical references and index.
Identifiers: Canadiana (print) 20210364246 | Canadiana (ebook) 20210364262 |
ISBN 9781487541606 (cloth) | ISBN 9781487541637 (EPUB) |
ISBN 9781487541620 (PDF)
Subjects: LCSH: Livestock – Breeding – History. | LCSH: Human-animal relationships – History.
Classification: LCC SF105 .D46 2022 | DDC 636.08/209–dc23

We wish to acknowledge the land on which the University of Toronto Press operates. This land is the traditional territory of the Wendat, the Anishnaabeg, the Haudenosaunee, the Métis, and the Mississaugas of the Credit First Nation.

University of Toronto Press acknowledges the financial support of the Government of Canada, the Canada Council for the Arts, and the Ontario Arts Council, an agency of the Government of Ontario, for its publishing activities.

Canada Council for the Arts
Conseil des Arts du Canada

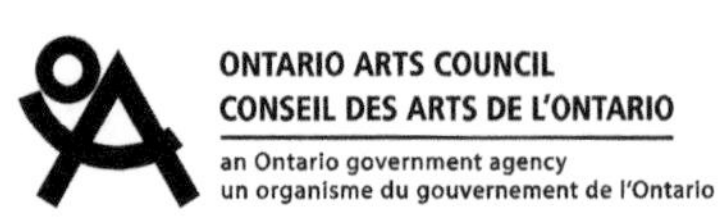

Funded by the Government of Canada
Financé par le gouvernement du Canada
Canadä

Contents

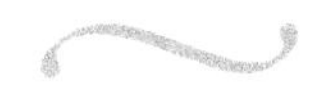

MADE TO ORDER

The Designing of Animals

Introduction

One day in 1880 a number of cattlemen wandered around the barns at Bow Park, a Shorthorn breeding farm in Ontario, Canada. While looking over the animals, they discussed the problems of the times that faced this important beef breed. In the middle of their conversation, the men stopped for a moment by the stall of a bull, Fourth Duke of Clarence. The bull "had a majestic step and a wonderfully expressive head, and while looking out of his box he would greet [the farm manager, John Hope,] with a low bellow and then lick[ed] his hand," one visitor reminisced many years later, noting as well that a very close bond, based on respect, existed between man and animal. "There was a [marvellous] relationship betwixt the two." The Shorthorn trade for Canadian cattle in the United States had taken a strange turn by the late 1870s, and the men had gathered to thrash out the problem. The present market conditions demanded red cattle only, regardless of quality. All breeding bulls at Bow Park were, subsequently, red; the Fourth Duke being the lone exception. A rich roan, he was valuable because he produced mostly reds. While the men agreed, "you had to suit your market," they talked over what should or could be done, with respect to breeding plans put in place for the long run. The farm manager believed that, for the time being, the value of young red bulls would be strong, but the stress on red was not likely to endure. Would the breeding for red at present lead to the ruination of the Shorthorn breed in the future? That was the fundamental issue at hand. "The red craze [might be at] its height and [while] all ... efforts were to produce cattle of this color," the men thought it was a poor way to breed good stock. "The red craze ha[d] produced a lot of paper-skinned animals."[1]

This story introduces the fact that the breeding of animals reflects the impact of many complex matters. The 1880 discussion on Shorthorn breeding indicates some which will be enlarged upon in this book;

namely, the importance of the American market to how breeding proceeds, the significance of colour in breeding aims, and aspects of the animal/human relationship. *Made to Order* explains these factors and other breeding concerns as well in relation to both animals and society in North America and Europe over the past three centuries. The book does so by focusing on three overview topics; namely how breeding methodology evolved, what characterized the aims of breeding, and the way structures were put in place to regulate the occupation. Aims, money, societal structures, various attitudes to animals and their uses, as well as breeding methodology, with its practical and science axis, are organized within those three topics. The complex narratives found in the topics, resulting from an intertwining of such aspects, take on broader meaning when viewed as separate parts of the one larger story, namely that relating to animal breeding. I believe that a deeper understanding of animal breeding can be had from an appreciation of it as being a composite of separate, albeit intertwined histories.

It becomes evident, for example, that historical animal breeding has a more multi-faceted nature than first meets the eye. By structuring the book around an overview attitude to themes that span species and culture, rather than around a specific breed or nation, I also demonstrate that, for at least several hundred years, animal breeding has been not just complicated by persisting factors but also many-sided in surprisingly similar ways across species, geography, and time. Animal breeding history is fascinating, and I hope this analysis of three fundamental features of it will make some of its numerous patterns, and equally important their implications for the whole, better understood. By looking at breeding theory and method (section one), in conjunction with efforts at improvement through selection aims (section two), and the dynamics of marketing within a pedigree structure (section three), *Made to Order* explains patterns in historical animal breeding. Below I provide some detail on specific subjects found in the book, and also enlarge on how its contents are organized.

The first section, a discussion of breeding theory and methodology over centuries, has three chapters. They divide the subject into periods: Roman times to 1900; genetics and animal breeding, 1900–2000; and a chapter on developments in genetics and technology in relation to animal breeding from roughly 1980 to the present. The story of the naturalist and geneticist relationship to the practical breeding of animals can be divided neatly into the three chapter divisions. They comprise, concisely, the historic trends within periods that characterize how one interfaced with the other and why. The first chapter introduces several topics or themes that will run through the whole section and also underlie or resonate through aspects of the rest of the book. Of primary significance is the viewing of environmental breeding in relation to improvement breeding. The historic approach to animal breeding (that is, up to at least 1800) rested on attempting to control environmental factors. The idea that animals could be changed via breeding would be critical to all Western breeding by the late eighteenth century, but the ethos behind environmental breeding would never completely die out.

Another major topic introduced in chapter 1, which will play a role in explanations about genetics and practical animal breeding methods throughout section one, is the growth of two different theories concerning how to view the process of heredity, views which in the end played a significant role in how breeding strategies or methods evolved. One theory (known as force theory) supported the concept that heredity was directed by an unknown force which need not be understood in order to breed properly. The second theory (known as cell theory but what I also call gene or genetic architecture theory) argued that hereditary material itself had to be identified in order to breed properly. I suggest that breeding methods cannot be properly appreciated outside the context of these two theories. An oscillation between the two theories occurred for naturalists (and later geneticists). No such oscillation arose in practical breeder thinking. Practical breeders always supported the force theory. The oscillation factor does much to explain how conflicts developed between geneticists in particular and practical breeders, a problem that has tantalized historians for some time. How has science related to the culture in animal breeding? Why did animal breeders seem to remain impervious to genetics for so long? Why do they still not adhere especially closely to propositions emanating out of genetics? We will see that practical breeders actually did and do follow principles emanating from genetics in many cases. It is the impact of the oscillation between the two theories by geneticists which made it appear that practical breeders remained unreceptive to information from genetics.

Chapter 2 of this section covers developments under Mendelism, population genetics, and quantitative genetics; that is roughly 1900 to 2000. Linkages between practical breeder theory over the late eighteenth and across the nineteenth century and other theories, particularly quantitative genetics, will be obvious. With the rise of Mendelism we see how the divisive patterns laid down over the late eighteenth and over the nineteenth centuries played themselves out. The cleavage led to the direct involvement of scientists in practical breeding and, in doing so, divided the breeding industry into a group where breeders were commercialized via corporate enterprise and one where breeders remained in charge. Patterns basic to that critical deviation became clearly evident. The third chapter, which is primarily focused on 1990 to 2020, assesses the effects of molecular genetics, genomics and its contingent technology, and lastly epigenetics on animal breeding. Theoretical foundations underlying quantitative genetics, it will be clear, would also be basic to a genomic approach to animal breeding and concurrently to genomic technology. Epigenetics suggests that there will not necessarily be a change in the future over that outlook.

In the second section I concentrate on certain aims driving breeding and provide examples of what such aims entailed. Methodology must be directed to an end, and here we see that endless possibilities present themselves. Perceptions concerning what to breed for have drastically affected the shape and character of pet, hobbyist, and farm animals across species (and the various breeds within them) over time and different countries since at least the late eighteenth century. I found that by focusing on various breeding aims I could, for one thing, show how complicated the simple idea of improvement could be. This section also has three chapters. The first chapter (chapter 4) reviews aspects of breeding in relation to specialization of purpose or use. Should animals be expected to serve several purposes equally well (for example, supply quantities of beef and milk)? Or should one be sacrificed at least to some degree for the advancement of the other? If a single use is emphasized in cattle breeding, milk for example, the second purpose could be served in a by-product way. Male calves could be marketed for meat, even if not in the economic way that specialized beef-bred cattle are. Sometimes specialization for one purpose simply ended any production of the other. Such is the case today in egg-laying chickens. It is not worth raising male chicks from egg-laying strains for meat. They are killed at birth.

Breeding animals for single use, however, would have other ramifications. For one thing, the gender of the people caring for certain stock shifted from female to male. For another, attitudes towards animals readjusted in interesting ways, with the masculinization of aspects of agriculture. The sense that dairy cows were machines gathered momentum in North America and the Netherlands as well as other parts of Europe, but always in relation to the level of commercialization and the increased domination of men in the industry. By the 1970s, long after North Americans (with dairying in the hands of men) argued that cows were machines, farmers in the Netherlands began to see it that way. Dairy cattle breeders were advised after that time to view the animals as objects that made milk. Comments such as "There's no room for pet cows in modern farming" and breeding work "is aimed at … the commercial farmers, the dairymen who earn money by producing milk" were increasingly common.[2]

The second chapter of this section (chapter 5) looks at the role that selection for colour played in animal breeding. Is the desire for a certain colour simply a matter of taste, or preference? Were economic factors part of the story, and, if so, how? We will see that, like any other breeding aim, the reasons for selecting for a certain colour were complicated, and usually made sense within the framework of a number of factors. Rarely was it simply a matter of taste. Sport, genetics, and industry structure were a few of the underlying factors driving the choice to focus on (or avoid) a certain colour. The third chapter (chapter 6) assesses the authenticity factor, namely trueness to historic type, in selective breeding. Since authenticity breeding often means reversion away from improvement breeding in favour of environmental breeding, it is particularly interesting to study. There are other reasons for looking carefully at authenticity breeding. What, for example, can we learn about why people breed, what motivates them? Does authenticity breeding explain anything about an ongoing dichotomy: did people breed for love of animals or for monetary gain?

Improvement breeding, when in conjunction with ever more invasive commercialization, fuelled the dichotomy, thereby muddying the water. Comments such as the following about money and its relationship to love might be common, but they are clearly ambiguous when seen within the broader context of the breeding environment and rise of commercialism.[3] "It may be argued that the breeders of pure-bred [animals] are in the business for the money they make out of it," a Canadian cattle breeder noted in 1899. But this is not so, he argued, contending that it was love of the work that motivated purebred breeders.[4] Monetary matters were secondary. Similar arguments could be found in American attitudes to the market in relation to dog breeding in the mid-twentieth century.[5] Breeders still contend that they love the occupation, pursue it because they enjoy it, and hope that they are creating something worthwhile. But what ultimately is the relationship of money to breeding, or to the motivation to breed? The complicated ideals behind authenticity breeding, as revealed in this book, make it evident that both love and money played a role in breeding. While monetary gain often did play the major role, in authenticity breeding the love was clearly there. Economic factors were not the only ones which might direct breeding.

In the third section I address the issue of how to regulate and organize breeding, and do so by reviewing the way structures, mostly those connected to the purebred system, affected markets, which in turn skewed breeding. At the heart of the matter were pedigrees and their standards. The two chapters of this section not only make the point that pedigrees played a significant role in market conditions but also show how and why that was the case. Pedigrees, not breeding ideology or method, for example, often created or even destroyed breeds, and in the process defined their relative value. Pedigrees themselves could be bought and sold when either legitimately or fraudulently attached to certain animals. A review of the global Arabian horse market ties together various issues in the sections. The powerful interplay between purity and authenticity would be directed by pedigrees. Dreams of perfection, often defined by globally accepted pedigrees, became intertwined with ancient breeding principles that rested on perpetuation of type. The panorama of human thought is impressive in the Arabian horse story.

Approaching the topic of animal breeding within a framework of three overarching factors helps overcome the sense that historical animal breeding often seems to reflect a sense of myth and legend. I believe it is that sense in recent times which has helped attract a number of scholars wishing to dispel the mistiness surrounding the subject. Because animal breeding has been shaped by attitudes to the natural world, science, culture, human-animal bonds, markets and trade, the production of food, attempts to create beauty, and the need for companionship, a proliferation of diverse material on animal-related matters has appeared. *Made to Order* adds to this historiography. The book analyses the subject by reorganizing information on a broad range of topics that I have collected over the past twenty years. A considerable amount of new research went into enriching my story. How the book fits into the broader academic literature concerning animals, breeding, society, and time frame, however, is worth (at least) briefly outlining.

With respect to the first section, the history of breeding itself, the tendency of historians has been, first, to look only at the early twentieth century and, second, not to study animals at all, but rather to concentrate on the breeding of plants.[6] There are, of course, important exceptions which do deal with animals in that period and later as well, the most recent being Bert Theunissen's *Beauty or Statistics: Practice and Science in Dutch Livestock Breeding, 1900–2000* (2020).[7] An assessment of eugenics and its relationship to both practical animal breeders and geneticists has commanded interest, again with a focus on the early twentieth century.[8] Genetics and animal breeding after 1960 have received little attention, relatively speaking, from historians, although that situation is rapidly changing, Theunissen's *Beauty or Statistics* being a prime example.[9]

With respect to the theme of the second section, the varying implications of selection aims, this topic has only recently become a major concern to scholars. It is dealt with as one aspect of the purebred dog fancy by Michael Worboys, Julie-Marie Strange, and Neil Pemberton in their *The Invention of the Modern Dog: Breed and Blood in Victorian Britain* (2018). By far the most significant look at how one important selection aim operated, namely specialization, is Edmund Russell's *Greyhound Nation: A Coevolutionary History of England, 1200–1900* (2018). *Greyhound Nation* looks at specialization within the framework of human-animal coexistence. The book also addresses environmental breeding in relation to improvement breeding (a subject that arises in all three sections of *Made to Order*).

The theme of the third section in this book, regulation of breeding as seen through pedigrees, has commanded little attention from historians as to any widespread or varying impact, beyond the simple recognition that pedigrees had economic implications. The interconnected topic of pedigrees, breeding, and markets has not been studied in much detail, but there is evidence that that situation is changing.[10] Rebecca Woods's *The Herds Shot around the World: Native Breeds and the British Empire, 1800–1900* (2017) assesses international affairs relating to the fortunes of cattle and sheep breeds within that general framework. How pedigrees in particular fit with rising attitudes to eugenics or class consciousness has been more important to scholarly research than an appraisal of actual breeding and markets, and therefore still tends to dominate work on the nature of purebred breeding and pedigree keeping.[11] The way that pedigrees drive markets as well as skew breeding itself takes centre stage in this book.

I think it is worth including a short discussion about the nature of the sources I used and why I used them. There are three points about sources that are worth looking at, ones I consider important to any study of historical animal breeding. To begin with, I believe an interdisciplinary approach to the study of animal breeding is critical. I suggest that an increased sense of interconnected and more interdisciplinary research greatly enhances animal studies. For me, though, reading only the history of science and not science itself fails to provide the research needed to make a book truly an interdisciplinary study. Actual science articles enrich an appreciation of what scientists (and earlier naturalists) offered practical breeders. It becomes more evident whether or not any scientists' (or naturalists') thoughts, theories, or methods would be useful to practical breeders. Quantitative genetics in relation to cattle breeding, for example, cannot be understood properly without reading at least some of the publications of Jay Lush, Sewall Wright, and R.A.

Fisher. There are excellent secondary sources which outline and clearly describe the theories of these scientists, but a deeper understanding of the implications behind secondary sources only emerges from a reading of what the three men actually wrote. I would argue further that one reason there is so little academic history on late twentieth- and early twenty-first-century practical breeding comes from the fact that science is rarely used in the service of history. Because all modern breeding at least reflects aspects of quantitative genetics, a clear appreciation of that science and its evolution seems to me to be mandatory for a history of modern animal breeding.

Second, I avoid the tendency to compartmentalize the subject of domestic animal breeding into that relating to farm animals (cattle and work horses, for example), and that relating to hobbyist animals (dogs, and to some degree Arabian and Thoroughbred horses). Focusing on one and ignoring the other fundamentally weakens any true appreciation for the history and culture of animal breeding. Such an approach restricts the breadth of both primary and secondary sources used in research. Hobbyist breeders articulated practical breeder thoughts more clearly (and more often) than did farm animal breeders. That situation makes dog and fancy chicken breeder commentary particularly significant when it comes to assessing how hereditary laws were viewed by practical breeders and how these people saw science in relation to practice. Literature by hobbyists can also be surprisingly astute. Examples abound. Collie breeder William Mason's reinterpretation of purebred breeding, in light of Mendelian theory early in the twentieth century, is a classic example of how primary source, hobbyist views can provide a window into the general world of practical breeders, as well as into their appreciation of science. An enriched view on the strategies of pre-eighteenth-century breeding (therefore environmental breeding) can be had from reading the primary source work of John Walsh (aka Stonehenge) on mid-nineteenth-century Greyhound breeding. Contrasting these hobbyist views with those proposed by cattle breeders can be especially rewarding. In other words, by doing research into hobbyist and agricultural breeding combined, we can understand more about all animal breeding.

The third point I wish to address is the need to separate, if at all possible, the views of expert practical breeders (generally agricultural college people, government officials, and purebred breeders) from general practical breeders. While all practical breeders supported the force theory, the two groups did not hold similar views on important issues. That situation is particularly evident when it comes to agricultural breeding, because often farmers seemed to have a better basic understanding of certain breeding principles than did the experts and purebred breeders. Unfortunately, the voice of the practical farmer, as opposed to the expert or purebred breeder, is often hard to hear. Any documentation that records non-expert practical breeder views is, therefore, invaluable. There are three sources that can be useful when trying to deal with this problem. Government documents sometimes set out in detail what farmers thought about expert attitudes to breeding. One example can be found in discussion arising from the late nineteenth-century stallion legislation issue, where general horsemen expressed views on the nature of heredity. Second, letters by farmers to agricultural journals from the late nineteenth to the early twentieth century are also helpful, and can reveal how farmers reacted to the advice constantly being bombarded at them by experts and purebred breeders. And third, when it comes to modern times, chat lines on the Internet are indispensable, not just for practical breeder opinion but also for the history of animal breeding from the 1960s to the present. In some ways these Internet chats are the only sources we have about late twentieth-century animal breeding from a practical point of view. Many of the people discussing issues after 2010 on the Internet lived through the period, as early as the 1960s, when concerns triggering the present dialogue actually arose. I am surprised, actually, at how under-utilized this source tends to be.

Made to Order deals with a number of specialized subjects, and while I attempted to handle them in a user-friendly way without the use of jargon, it was impossible to completely remove language that might be foreign to some readers. I explain terms in the text and try to stay with simple (and single) definitions, but it seemed advisable to add a glossary at the end. Readers, therefore, can easily look up terminology that is new to them. This can be especially useful when terms and issues re-emerge in later parts of the book.

Readers who would like to know what breeding entails, from the point of view of at least three of the many separate spokes that explain it, should get a grasp from this book of patterns which over time have become entangled with each other. The broad range of sources used to produce *Made to Order* helps show how complicated the factors behind evolving patterns could be. Readers, I hope, will be able to formulate useful views on basic subjects which, in spite of the considerable amount of literature around animals, often remain hidden or at least unexplained with any clarity. Animal breeding is an ancient human practice, and there is little to say it won't continue to be important in the future, or that historic patterns in it will change. Its past and present tell us much about how human thinking, theorizing, and evolving approaches characterize our interaction with all natural processes.

Some patterns that persist in today's breeding seem almost nonsensical (intense inbreeding in dogs, for example, as a result of pedigree registries having a narrow genetic base), but when seen against how such patterns evolved, as well as how widespread they have always been, it becomes apparent that convictions emanating from the past are still very much with us, and as a result explain the present. Perhaps this book will help us achieve a better understanding of modern breeding dynamics in many parts of the world.

SECTION ONE

How to Breed Animals: Theory and Method, Eighteenth to Twenty-First Century

Chapter One

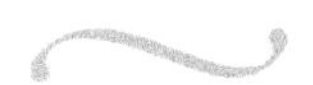

Animal Breeding Practices and Methods from Roman Times to 1900

This first section lays the groundwork of the story of historical animal breeding by outlining how breeding methods evolved.[1] Because methods and theories tended to develop within the world of agricultural animal breeding, much of the section emphasizes breeding and the conflicts that arose over it within that environment. It is important to note that the methods and underlying theories utilized for farm animals would play themselves out in the world of pet, hobbyist, and (one could add) laboratory breeding, as will be evident in later sections. The more apparent economic implications of farm animal breeding, and its vital relation to the welfare of the state and society, probably explain why broadly held human attitudes to the breeding of domestic animals were inclined to develop within the framework of agricultural needs. The situation also explains why science became involved with how effective methods of selection were in the breeding of food animals. Two opposing groups quickly became evident under these conditions: practical breeders and scientists. What shaped methods and theories and the conflicts arising between the groups would be the position taken over the centuries by the practical breeders, as opposed to that taken by naturalists (later scientists, meaning geneticists), about what heredity meant and how one should approach it. While the seeds for conflict were laid down as early as the eighteenth century, disagreements did not crystallize into open discord until the twentieth century when geneticists confronted the combined group of practical breeders (purebred breeders and their supporters, as well as general farmers). The groundwork for the subject of breeding strategies is addressed in this chapter by assessing how methods and practices evolved from Roman times until the advent of genetics, namely the rediscovery of Mendel's laws in 1900.

Breeding before the Eighteenth Century

Until the end of the seventeenth century, generally speaking only one group, that is the practical breeders, addressed animal breeding. Selection strategies for practical purposes received serious European attention as early as Roman times. The first known articulated principle had been set out by Varro, who hinted at an important breeding tool: progeny testing. Offspring should be used to judge the breeding quality of the parents.[2] In the first century AD and a hundred years after Varro, Columella enlarged on the subject in his twelve-volume *De re rustica*.[3] The breeding strategies set out by classical writers were all based on their attitude to what drove the process of heredity. They saw heredity as a phenomenon which resulted from the effects of the environment, not from some innate biological material within living things. After the fall of Rome and until the early eighteenth century, practical breeders continued to be influenced by this concept, which argued that what animals ate and the environment in which they ate it affected what the creatures became.[4] Under these conditions, practical continental European and British breeders used varying breeding strategies to counteract the effects of environment on heredity in order to maintain the quality of animals rather than improve them.[5] Throughout the book I refer to this approach, and the subsequent methods adopted in light of it, as environmental breeding.[6]

Attitudes to heredity did not attract the notice of a second group until the mid-eighteenth century, namely the naturalists. These people formed a mixed group of thinkers across Europe, from different intellectual backgrounds and training, who observed the natural world. Their commonality resulted from their desire to understand the dynamics behind all aspects of it, generally speaking by postulating and then testing theories. Naturalists' views on heredity up until that time had been irrevocably entangled with their opinions concerning generation (via conception, birth, and embryology).[7] Heredity as a process in its own right had been a foreign concept to them. They started to address the nature of heredity itself during the Enlightenment, and came to see it as a separate process, a vague but overall "force." In effect the naturalists had adopted what is known as force theory.

This new attitude influenced the thinking of the practical breeders. They interpreted the theory to mean that heredity could be detached from environmental factors. It was a profound reorientation, ultimately changing the motives behind practical breeder selection tactics. For breeders, force theory implied that heredity could be manipulated to advance human concerns. Under these conditions, the objectives of the practical breeders changed completely. They became focused on developing various strategies designed to bring about improvement of certain features in animals.[8] The conviction that quality was a maintenance issue, however, is a highly significant concept in animal breeding and did not die after that time.[9] (In modern terms this matter might be defined as the "nature versus nurture" dilemma.) Practical breeders would continue, however, to be interested only in results, not in the underlying dynamics behind those results.

Bakewellianism and Thoroughbred Horse Breeding

Methods designed by the practical breeders to bring about improvement within that theoretical framework developed quickly, and rested on the conviction that good breeding could proceed with no knowledge of underlying hereditary laws. Experience taught what systems brought desired results because only through experience could a breeder learn which selection strategies worked best to increase the ability of chickens to lay eggs, cows to give milk, cattle to develop good meat qualities, or horses to have greater speed or strength. Two particularly important methods, which both arose from that standpoint, took shape in England. The two methods would play an enormously important role in practical breeding systems over the nineteenth and twentieth centuries. The first evolved from a desire to make farm animals more uniform in type and better for agricultural production, and while many breeders probably contributed to the framing of the method, it is the British farmer Robert Bakewell (1725–1795) who gets the credit for its popularity.[10] While Bakewell himself wrote little about his breeding methods, letters of the Culley brothers, reports by agriculturalist Arthur Young, and a treatise by the breeder Sir John Sebright make it clear what Bakewell's principles were.[11] Fundamentally, these principles emanated from viewing the process of heredity through the lens of the force theory.

Bakewell's system was based on three primary premises. They were, first, inbreeding for type; second, equal emphasis on males and females (which were believed to contribute as much to offspring as males); and third, selection for both quality and vigour on the basis of the progeny test, meaning an animal's worth should be judged on the general quality of its offspring.[12] Inbreeding and offspring quality, to put it succinctly, were the cornerstones of his method. Bakewell tended to emphasize males in his inbreeding programs. Since a male provides half the hereditary input to a herd or population, Bakewell could assess resulting changes in a herd more effectively by keeping track of sires.

The acceptability of inbreeding, though, which Bakewell encouraged, was probably the most critical contribution he made to future animal breeding. Sir John Sebright believed that to be the case. In 1809 he wrote: "Mr. Bakewell had certainly the merit of destroying the absurd prejudices which formerly prevailed against breeding from animals, between whom there was any degree of relationship," and expanded as follows: "had this opinion been universally acted upon, no one could have been said to be possessed of a particular breed, good or bad."[13] In other words, before Bakewell's time, the best breeders, perhaps few in number, had always practised inbreeding. Bakewell's system was aimed at creating lines that bred truly over generations. He intended to establish a type of animal that would be consistent and recognizable as a distinct "breed," and he hoped to bring about gradual improvement of that fixed type over generations.

It has been argued that Bakewell and his fellow farm breeders were the first to look at the inheritance factor involving improvement in terms of groups or populations rather than individuals.[14] Volume was especially important to Bakewell, because he saw breeding as a tool to rapidly augment food production for Britain's growing population, a trend which worried many and culminated in the famous 1798 treatise of Thomas Malthus, who theorized that the food supply could not keep up with population growth. Although no accurate figures existed before 1801 on the actual population of England and Wales, many individuals in the eighteenth century were aware that the number of people was growing at a disproportionate rate. Clearly Bakewell recognized that there would be an ever larger market for food supplies, particularly meat, as this trend progressed. He was interested in stamping type (therefore creating "breeds"), because he wanted to standardize type in order to sustain higher levels of production. Bakewellianism was developed to work with assumed hereditary laws – laws that seemed evident from breeding experience – in order to achieve the objectives of breeding; namely better, more uniform farm animals in greater volume. Bakewell recognized the value of livestock breeders working together as a group, and in 1783 formed an organization, the Dishley Society, to advance their interests. The Society could be said to be the forerunner of the various breed associations established in Europe and North America over the late nineteenth century.

The second breeding method resulted from the development of the Thoroughbred horse. Like Bakewell, the horse breeders accepted heredity as an unknown force that could be manipulated. But Thoroughbred horse breeding varied from Bakewell's method in five critical ways. First, Thoroughbred horse breeding emphasized the input of males over females. The system was based on crossbreeding, namely the crossing of Arabians on local horses – classically Arabian stallions on local mares, although later DNA testing has shown that Arabian females played a significant role in the makeup of early Thoroughbreds.[15] The crosses were considered to be "thoroughly bred," and therefore labelled "Thoroughbred." Second, selection should be based on the ancestral background of an animal, rather than its offspring. Third, the quality of the individual horse, not the population it fitted into, should influence breeding decisions. Fourth, inbreeding was avoided. And fifth, public pedigree keeping was central to the system because of concern with ancestry breeding. The General Stud Book, established as early as 1791 by James Weatherby, recorded pedigrees for these horses. Pedigree keeping introduced concepts of purity and status to animals.[16] From the beginning, the elite members of society (royalty and the nobility) were the principal breeders and that fact meant their class views shaped and coloured horse-breeding philosophy. The cultural and social impressions that arose from these associations would be significant over the years.

Both methods were designed to provide improvement by taking into account what past experience had taught breeders; namely the contradictory effects that inbreeding, outcrossing, and crossbreeding strategies had on the resulting progeny. As far back as Roman times, they had understood that inbreeding produced uniformity, and also that it could reduce the vigour and fertility of plants and animals. The crossing of inbred lines, or outcrossing, they had learned, would bring a return of both vigour and fertility, sometimes in a most spectacular way. First-generation crosses of this nature were known to show advanced improvement. There were problems, however, in pursuing this type of selection as a prominent breeding method. The improved state of the first-generation progeny would not endure into another generation. Breeders came to recognize that the outcrossed progeny of the two inbred lines, while it might be better than the mean of the parent lines, would not breed truly to its improved state.[17] (Naturalists – and subsequently geneticists – would later describe this specific type of improvement as hybrid vigour.) Probably more commonly, breeders used the outcrossing method in a different fashion, namely by mating animals from non-inbred families, but, by always working within the same type, thereby restricting selection choices. The second form of outcrossing produced results, although in a somewhat weakened way, similar to the first; potentially superior progeny that would not breed truly. Breeders also utilized crossbreeding, meaning the mating of animals belonging to different breeds or types. While the strategy could yield good progeny, like any kind of outcrossing, that progeny would not breed truly.

Up to the early eighteenth century, breeding methods might have taken these features into account, but they had been used to counteract the effects of the environment. French breeders, for example, often chose to rely on outcrossing non-related families or even crossbreeding different types in order to neutralize environmental effects.[18] German farmers, on the other hand, were more likely to use inbreeding as a tool to control environmental impact.[19] They believed uniformity provided hereditary strength. European sheep breeders tended to share the German view: namely that avoidance of crossbreeding in particular preserved power against environmentally induced factors.[20]

Breeders in the eighteenth century devised more structured, albeit different, approaches to working with these known complex patterns and to neutralizing the dangers that came with excessive inbreeding, outcrossing, or crossbreeding in order to achieve improvement. Bakewell's system focused on inbreeding, and intense inbreeding at that. He planned to capitalize on the benefits (namely uniformity) it offered, and to minimize its dangers. Selection and the progeny test made it possible to identify good animals. It was the percentage of good and strong offspring over bad and weakened that defined the parent as a superior breeder. Good offspring that withstood inbreeding were often bred back to that parent. Avoidance of inbreeding by Thoroughbred horse breeders meant they were not faced with inbreeding difficulties, but the unpredictability that came from crossbreeding (as a result of input from Arabians) or even mild outcrossing (the mating of unrelated families within the evolving Thoroughbred pool) confronted them. Thoroughbred horse breeders believed that that problem would be overcome by relying on ancestry breeding, namely the past performance of particular but unrelated males recorded in pedigrees. The input of quality ancestors via their descendants might not guarantee success, but it did enhance the odds of getting good results. The challenge of working with this interplay of inbreeding, outcrossing, and crossbreeding would dominate all future breeding methodology, whether it related to practical strategies, naturalist breeding, or genetic selection.

Naturalist Approaches and the Rise of Purebred Breeding

Naturalist thinking might have shifted the focus of the practical breeder towards improvement, but by the end of the eighteenth century practical breeder activity began, in turn, to influence naturalist thinking.

Naturalist awareness of practical breeding originated with a simple interest in the variation that breeder selection strategies brought about in animals. The deviation as to type fascinated naturalists. At first, they took no interest in the breeding process that had brought about such changes: the breeding results alone commanded their attention. In 1745 the French mathematician and astronomer Pierre-Louis de Maupertuis (1698–1759), for example, had noted that artificial selection was capable of altering domestic animals and plants, and he wondered if natural selection could be powerful enough to cause the development of new species.[21] It was not long, however, before naturalists wondered if their own breeding experiments might enlighten them on the way the heredity force theory operated.

In 1751 Swedish botanist Carl Linnaeus published a systematic discussion of plant hybrids – inbreeding and crossing inbred lines or strains, and even crossbreeding species. In effect Linnaeus founded what would subsequently be defined as the hybridist tradition. The first person to be credited with working with the hybrid breeding method was the German travel writer, historian, and geographer, J.G. Kölreuter, who published the work of his experiments in 1761.[22] Perhaps, naturalists increasingly postulated, not just the dynamics of hereditary factors but also the way species developed could be revealed through hybridist breeding exercises. Hybrid breeding would, as a consequence, soon become the favourite way to breed for experimental reasons and scientific analysis.[23] Naturalists, in effect, had become "breeders." By the end of the eighteenth century, then, two groups of breeders existed.

Experimenting naturalists initially focused on plant breeding in their inbreeding and outcrossing work in order to achieve variation in the offspring, a pattern most strongly seen in outcrossing inbred lines or from the crossbreeding of animal types with no relationship to each other. Deviation was what the experimenters were after. They did not want uniformity, and therefore avoided the breeding of "like to like" which resulted in true breeding lines or "breeds." No underlying laws would be revealed through such homogeneity. In the nineteenth century, when naturalists began in a limited way to experiment with animal breeding, they did so with the inbreeding and outcrossing of lines used by the experimental plant breeders, and for the same reasons. In 1819 Hungarian nobleman Count Festetics, for example, undertook hybridist experiments with animals, and subsequently wrote a treatise named "Hereditary Laws of Nature."[24] All experimental breeding was directed at understanding what lay behind the force theory, and therefore what drove the variation ultimately resulting in the rise of new species. Naturalists persisted in seeking deviation or variation in progeny which in turn were not intended for use in future breeding. Practical breeders remained concerned with the continuity found in breeds or true breeding lines.[25]

Early in the nineteenth century, patterns in practical breeding methodology shifted in significant ways. Purebred breeding was born. The new method developed from a fusion of Bakewellianism and Thoroughbred horse breeding. Its creation can be attributed to the work of one man, the English livestock breeder Thomas Bates. About 1800 he began to acquire Shorthorn cattle, bred by the Colling brothers on the basis of Bakewellian principles. Bates then followed a new breeding strategy in which he incorporated tenets of Thoroughbred horse breeding with Bakewell's strategies. Bates recognized that the horse-breeding system had proved to be a powerful marketing tool, with its emphasis on keeping publicly recorded pedigrees and the idea of purity. In his new system, Bates linked inbreeding, purity, and reliance on ancestry for breeding purposes together through the use of public pedigrees. He championed the registry that George Coates established for Shorthorns in 1822, and argued that it provided proof of inbreeding and therefore purity in the stock.[26]

His linkage of inbreeding with purity was new. Inbreeding for Bakewell had nothing to do with purity, and purity for horse breeders had nothing to do with inbreeding. The inbreeding linkage with purity embedded in all future purebred breeding brought with it different meanings to the Bakewellianism principle of inbreeding. Under Bakewell it meant primarily consistency of type; under Bates it did the same but also implied lack of contamination, a concept derived from the purity concerns of Thoroughbred horse breeders. Bates quickly attracted buyers among members of the landed aristocratic class in Britain, and American importers as well. His reputation as a brilliant breeder, but also a great promoter, grew ever more widespread.[27] Bates died in 1850, but his method lived on to dominate animal breeding methodology for improvement.

With the passage of time, it became increasingly obvious that many purebred breeders ceased to recognize that Bates's breeding system was not synonymous with Bakewellianism, or that the infiltration of Thoroughbred horse culture into farm breeding had brought about the expansion of an entirely new method, albeit one that still rested on the theoretical view that hereditary force could be manipulated without knowing what the dynamics of that force might be. When explaining the purebred method to farmers in North America, for example, editors of journals simply outlined Bakewell's principles, implying that they matched those of purebred breeding. Especially noticeable was their linkage of the keeping of public pedigrees with the Bakewellian system.[28] Bates's system, with its newly introduced Thoroughbred horse culture, also led to the critically declining influence of Bakewell's most important principles on breeding systems; namely, breeding by the progeny test with an emphasis on changes across populations.

The infusion of Thoroughbred horse culture into the method led in turn to the spread of complicated views which implied that quality in animals could be related to that in people. Purebred breeding provided a rationale for giving the concept of purity ethical and social implications, because, by providing apparent evidence of purity's value, it supported eugenics, which spread throughout societies around the world.[29] It should be noted, though, that it tended to be non-breeders, not breeders, who saw eugenics as part of animal breeding. Virtually nothing on eugenics as an underlying aspect of animal breeding appeared in literature devoted to farmers. Eugenics could be laughed at in the agricultural press, and farmers tended to take offence when eugenicists accused them of not adhering to eugenic principles in animal breeding. While it is undeniable that a linkage between societal and eugenic attitudes to animal breeding (through an emphasis on purity) evolved, for breeders the underlying power of "purity" remained consistency of type in animals, whether a result of selection via ancestry or selection via quality of offspring. Consistency of type meant marketing power.

Bates's strategy created cattle that were in demand, indicating that the system had economic implications. It enhanced the marketability of animals bred to its standards, and that factor drove the spread of the method's use, first in Britain, then in continental Europe and North America. By the late nineteenth century the method had become the most favoured strategy for improvement breeding throughout the Western world. Structures to support purebred breeding, namely breed associations and joint-purebred organizations, arose and effectively orchestrated ideas around how breeding should ideally proceed in most livestock industries. Purebred breeders promoted the method's value on the basis of endorsement from agricultural institutions and governments. The influence of the method on breeding would be profound: all breeding theory came to reflect its impact even if not all animals were purebred, and all breeding manifested the same concern that purebred breeders had with producing true lines.

While the literature addressing purebred breeding and its effects on both animals and humans is vast, for the purposes of this book four factors are particularly important. They are, first, when the science of genetics entered the world of agricultural breeding, purebred breeding was the most important type of practical improvement breeding.

Second, purebred breeding brought significant moves away from Bakewell's emphasis on offspring to judge the quality of an animal as well as his concern with improvement as a population issue. Third, the idea of purity took a more prominent role in the evaluation of quality in an animal. And fourth, the importance of monetary worth in breeding resulted in ever more important consequences. Critical implications would emerge from all these factors.

Cleavage in Naturalist Thinking: The Rise of Cell Theory and Biometry

During the period of purebred breeding expansion, important developments occurred in naturalist circles. A clear split between two factions evolved over how to study heredity. By 1860, while notions of heredity under the force theory remained in the minds of some, others began to conceptualize inheritance within a cell theory framework, meaning that some specific and potentially identifiable physical matter must lie behind the process of heredity.[30] (With the rise of genetics in 1900, cell theory, in effect, would become gene or genetic architecture theory.) Efforts to detect characteristics of the substance encouraged greater emphasis on experimental hybridist breeding. The rise of cell theory initiated a profound deviation in outlook concerning the nature of heredity between the naturalist group that supported it and practical breeders. Breeder views regarding heredity remained underpinned throughout the nineteenth and twentieth centuries by the force theory. Breeders believed that animals could be manipulated and changed without any real understanding of the dynamics behind the force.[31] Naturalists who continued to function within the force theory, then, shared a theoretical base with the practical breeders. It was a union that in the end would be profitable to both.

Conflict soon evolved not only between practical breeders and one naturalist faction but also between the naturalist sections themselves because of the theoretical split concerning force and cell theory. Troubles erupted when it became apparent that the two outlooks offered different ways of approaching Charles Darwin's views on evolution. Darwin had spent a great deal of time reading about the way artificial selection was practised by both experimental naturalists and practical breeders.[32] In his attempts to explain the process of natural selection, for example, Darwin had studied the hybridizing work of plant and animal breeders.[33] The cell theory naturalist group sought to understand the implications of Darwinism via experimental breeding and by using that same traditional hybridist method. They hoped to gain knowledge of how the physical material that directed heredity worked, and in the process elucidate the dynamics of evolution. Over the second half of the nineteenth century, much of biological research focused on explaining Darwin's evolutionary theory via this experimental breeding.

Inbreeding and outcrossing often came to be seen as a viable tool not just for the study of evolution but quite quickly as well for the improvement of agricultural plants. The Dutch plant physiologist Hugo de Vries (1848–1935), trained under German Julius von Sachs, was especially important to the trend of linking this form of breeding with experimentation designed to bring about better farming and to explain the dynamics of evolution.[34] Experimentation in evolutionary biology should be done at the agricultural experiment stations, he argued, because there were basic similarities between natural and artificial selection.[35] For biologists like de Vries, it was impossible to look at either separately from the other, and therefore any attempt to study one resulted in a study of the other. In a subtle way, biologists had moved themselves into the world of practical breeding. Under these conditions, the experimental methodology came increasingly to be seen as the educated way to practise artificial selection, and plant breeding by the method would dominate much of agricultural plant research at state-run institutions across North America by the late nineteenth century.[36] The same was true in Germany after the 1880s.[37]

The group of naturalists supporting the force theory took a different approach. These naturalists looked for an affinity between artificial and natural selection by focusing on how the shifting of animal types through the breeding of true lines could be extrapolated to patterns of evolution. Their views were not out of line with many aspects of Darwin's thinking. The apparent absence of inbreeding, outcrossing, or crossbreeding here (so different from hybridizing systems) fascinated Darwin, and he became interested in the effects of true line breeding on pigeons. A fancy pigeon breeder himself in 1856, Darwin corresponded with pigeon-breeding experts like John M. Eaton.[38] While pigeon breeders might have denounced both inbreeding and most particularly crossbreeding by this time (pigeon breeds had long been established by the mid-nineteenth century), they utilized these methods, albeit in a limited and underhanded way. Darwin looked beyond these practices and concentrated on the true line breeding emphasis of pigeon breeders, which he found important in the formulation of his theories around evolution. It particularly suited his analogy between artificial selection and natural selection, where inbreeding, outcrossing, and crossbreeding would only occur in a much weaker and more haphazard way.[39] The naturalists supporting force theory were inclined to be influenced by

Darwin's attitudes concerning what pigeon breeding meant in terms of evolution; namely that change under natural selection did not require extreme inbreeding and subsequently crossing. Furthermore, evolution could only be studied in terms of measuring population differences, not individual differences.

In an effort to understand natural selection in Darwin's terms, naturalists interested in force theory assessed variations in populations, not within individuals, using mathematics. The new statistical approach to heredity taken by these naturalists would come to be known as biometry, and was formally founded in 1886 by British geographer and mathematician Francis Galton. Born in 1822 and a cousin of Darwin, Galton studied medicine and mathematics at Cambridge University. Interested in geography in his early life, later he focused on the problem of inheritance via natural selection.[40] Consistent throughout his career, however, was his underlying fascination with quantification in patterns he studied. It was his idea that quantification could be applied to heredity which initiated biometry (and the journal *Biometrika* in order to pursue the study of biology through mathematics).[41] In effect, Galton invented biomathematics.[42]

He became particularly attracted to the study of human inheritance by way of mathematical measurements, and in 1883 coined the word "eugenics" to describe such research. When Galton addressed differences in people, he followed his quantitative approach, namely focusing on features that demonstrated quantitative inheritance (traits such as intelligence, height, etc.), characteristics which everyone inherited to varying degrees. Galton's method of looking at heredity via mathematical measurements attracted considerable widespread support after the publication in 1889 of his second book, *Natural Inheritance*.[43] The great statistician Karl Pearson and a marine biologist, W.F.R. Weldon, were both impressed with Galton's idea of using a statistical analysis to study patterns of inheritance. In the 1890s Pearson took over the crude statistical tools that Galton had developed and refined them to look in many ways like modern statistics.[44]

Biometry remained focused on natural, not artificial, selection and as such did not attempt to predict the outcome of any breeding strategy. It would be some time before the thinking behind biometry became applicable to artificial selection in animals for farm improvement, but few developments would be as important to future artificial selection theory emanating from science.[45] Animal breeders were primarily interested in quantitative traits: how much or how little of a characteristic a farm animal inherits as a result of certain breeding programs. Galton's affinity to the general outlook of animal breeders as to how heredity should be approached led him to an interest in their pedigree keeping. He amassed an immense amount of data generated by practical breeders, namely pedigrees of dogs, horses, and cattle. This linkage between naturalist and practical breeders through pedigrees makes an understanding of Galton's theorizing in relation to breeder thinking tantalizing. Was Galton directed by breeder theories, or were breeders directed by Galton theories?

Galton's reasoning in his ancestral law in particular bore a strong resemblance to that behind the thinking of at least some practical breeders. The similarities in views could be so stunning that one is forced to ask how much interplay actually took place between them. Galton put forward his law (initially formed by him in 1865 but not brought to true fruition until 1897) in "The Average Contribution of Each Several Ancestor to the Total Heritage of the Offspring," published in the *Proceedings of the Royal Society* in 1897. The law stated "that the two parents contribute between them on the average one half of the total inheritance of the offspring; the four grandparents one quarter," etc. "Furthermore," Galton added, "it is reasonable to believe that the contributions of parents to children are in the same proportion as those of the grandparents to the parents."[46] Pedigrees, then, explained how the hereditary input of ancestors could be understood. It was a matter of percentages in relation to generations. Galton believed his law was of vital importance to stock breeders, but some had already arrived at the same conclusion as early as the 1870s, either on their own or as a result of Galton's early thinking.[47]

All purebred breeders by that time believed that pedigrees (which are actually simply charts), and especially the attention to ancestry found in pedigrees, were important to understanding how heredity worked.[48] By the 1870s, however, a few (and not necessarily just purebred breeders) had gone on to analyse information in pedigrees more carefully. For these breeders, pedigrees acted as a critical selection device because they showed the hereditary input of ancestors to an individual in a generational way. Hereditary characteristics which that animal would pass on to its progeny could be appreciated, therefore, as a proportional issue. A significant example of this theoretical approach could be seen in one practical breeder's carefully constructed charts, based on pedigree, which were designed to explain how a percentage ancestry linkage could work.

American fancy chicken breeder I.K. Felch argued that by recombining the blood of an original breeding pair from different mating combinations over generations of their descendants, the heredity of the original pair could be regenerated in various blends. One could, therefore, inbreed (or line breed, according to his definition of the term) forever.[49] No outside blood need be introduced.[50] With careful selection, Felch could shift the hereditary makeup of the group he desired to work with, by changing the relative input of either original parent. By selecting only within that framework – that is, descendants of the foundation pair – he could ensure uniformity and also the maintenance of consistency. He concluded as follows: "As long as you can create groups representing half of the blood of each of the original Adam and Eve of your flock as reservoirs from which you can draw new blood for your mating … each group of chicks will show a change in their blood from that of their sires and dams. That is the secret of inbreeding."[51] As Felch put it, "We can mix the blood of our birds as easily as we mix paints that give us different tints of color."[52] His ideas and charts would be quoted and requoted (and sometimes presented with a few modifications that really were "little more than a steal")[53] throughout his life and after his death in 1918 at the age of eighty-four, even though momentous changes were shaking the world of hereditary science and practice by that time.[54]

While the theory of consistency in relation to documented ancestral percentage variations of inbreeding, the basis of Felch's breeding ideas, showed striking commonalities with Francis Galton's ancestral law, the timing of Galton's and Felch's views makes it difficult to establish whether one influenced the other, which way that went, or if the attitudes were arrived at independently. In his *The Breeding and Management of Poultry*, published in 1877, Felch spoke of "a natural law." He could have been simply referring to the force theory which drove all practical breeding, but he seemed to mean a specific "law," implying something more focused in impact. He argued: "If … breeders would adopt this plan of breeding and would keep a record, they would then see … how beautifully all these things are governed by a natural law."[55] Felch did not define what he meant by "a natural law," so it is not evident whether or not he had been influenced by developments in the naturalist world after Darwin's time. Apparently, though, calculating inbreeding ratios worked for the chicken breeder attempting to restrict and control hereditary input, while the utilization of a similar system proved useful to the naturalist at the same time.

A clearer example of the direct linkage of Galton's ancestral law with practical breeding, or that an interplay existed between them, can be found in the late nineteenth-century work of the English purebred Basset Hound breeder Everett Millais. In fact Millais's breeding and theories, as set out in his *The Theory and Practice of Rational Breeding* published in 1889, formed the basis of Galton's evidence to support his ancestral law. Everett Millais worked out charts showing effects of inbreeding and the outcross practice of mating unrelated families over generations within the Basset Hound breed. The important factor here was pedigrees: they worked naturally with Millais's purebred Basset Hound breeding and were helpful to the naturalist Galton when formulating theories. While Millais did not see a breeding system as enclosed in the same terms that Felch did (Millais believed in limited outcrossing and subsequent breeding over generations to remove undesired aspects of the outcross), he did argue that heredity could be calculated by assessing generational percentage charts, as had Felch. Millais went on until his death in 1896 publishing articles that further described his breeding theories in dog journalism.[56]

Such was the fractured and confusing situation with respect to how heredity was viewed by practical breeders and naturalists at the end of the nineteenth century. Cataclysmic changes, which would affect both groups, were just over the horizon.

Chapter Two

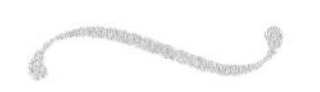

Mendelism, Quantitative Genetics, and Animal Breeding, 1900–2000

The birth of Mendelian genetics in 1900, with the rediscovery of Mendel's two laws of genetics, changed the whole picture. Gregor Mendel, a Moravian monk, had worked with the standard hybridizing (that is inbreeding and subsequently outcrossing) method as early as 1865. In modern terminology, he established two laws: first, when the gametes (or reproductive cells) form, the gene pairs separate (each unit of the pair is either recessive or dominant); and second, genes are both immutable and act independently (a view that subsequently has become somewhat modified). While it has been argued that Mendel only attempted to find new varieties by hybridizing existing ones, not to prove the existence of laws of genetics in any generalized way, in effect he did establish genetic laws and in the process invented a more controlled approach to research breeding. After 1900 his rediscoverers saw the method as a way to explore how Mendel's hereditary laws actually worked.[1]

Mendelian experimentation received the lion's share of research aid after 1900, and while plants continued to dominate the work, a number of studies were conducted on chickens, designed to assess deviations in colour, leg and wing shape, etc. Even though such research was largely funded by academic institutions in service to agriculture, it had little or nothing to do with increasing farm productivity.[2] The very interest of government in funding genetic studies within agricultural institutions, however, paved the way for a future refocus: namely a shift from breeding in order to understand genetic laws and therefore evolution to developing new breeding methods to achieve agricultural improvement.[3]

Practical breeders were fascinated by these developments, and almost from the beginning of Mendelism tried to see how the new information fitted with standard breeding practices. A good example of this can be seen in the writings of the important British Rough Collie dog breeder William Mason. It is impossible to think that Mason, a dog journalist, was not aware of Millais's theories and through him of Galton's ancestral law. Mason saw the advent of Mendelism in 1900 as profoundly important to animal breeding strategies, particularly because the new science completely undermined the theoretical base of Galton's ancestral law. What had made pedigrees important to both animal breeders and Galton's law was the belief that pedigrees provided correct evidence of hereditary input. That clearly could no longer be argued, because pedigrees, under Mendelian laws, did not account for recessive inheritance.

Mason wrote a series of articles in his *Collie Folio* about science and the breeding problem between 1908 and 1912. In these he clearly questioned not only the acceptance of Galton's ancestral law but also its utilization in specializing for purity. Furthermore, Mason questioned the assumption that any form of purity resulted from ancestral breeding. His remarks are worth quoting because they reveal how perceptive a practical breeder could be with respect to both Mendelism and Galton's theories. In January of 1908 he wrote an article entitled "Mendel's Theory."

> We had had no discovery in the principles of heredity that may compare with it since "The Origin of Species" and it will touch practical interests more closely than that landmark of philosophy. One's first thought is how glad Darwin would be were he alive ... Incidentally, the whole conception of what is meant by a pure breed has been altered. The new knowledge will enable the scientific grower to get a pure stock by crossing with stocks once thought impure, and this gives to the new variety at any time that it may be required all the strength of the mongrel without the least impairing its pure character.

We cannot yet use Mendel's law to improve animals but maybe we will be able to shortly, he added.[4] In September of 1911 he took up the story again in the *Collie Folio* under the title of "The Elusive Breeding Problem – Pedigree."

> In these days of Stud Book, pedigree stock – by which is implied animals of which the lineage can be traced back for some generations in these important volumes – is always regarded as more valuable than stock not so endowed. The possession of a Stud, Herd, or Flock Book is considered to enhance the value of the breed, and its formation is usually the first step in a systematical [*sic*] effort to breed to a definite type ... Although

> a pedigree animal is, broadly speaking, of greater value than one minus this adjunct, the new knowledge all tends to show us that undue importance may easily be attached to the possession of a string of names of this nature ... It is questionable if modern breeders as a whole do as well in their efforts to breed to type with a Stud Book at their backs, as their predecessors who had not this aid in the early and middle part of the last century.[5]

In June of 1912 Mason continued to assess the implications of Mendelism in relation to Galton, purity as consistency, and the value of looking at breeding groups over individuals. In the article entitled "The Elusive Breeding Problem – Purity," he wrote:

> The term "purity" as pursued by breeders receives new significance in the light of Mendel's discoveries. It used to be thought that "pure" stock was only obtained after generations of unions of like to like – that, in fact, the longer the pedigree the purer the race. Yet now we see that length of pedigree has very little to do with the matter. The recessive characters segregated out in the second generation from a cross are always pure. Purity means homogeneity in the units in the germ cells in respect to any given character. We must in future consider individuals from the standpoint of the units they bear rather than judge them by the actual appearance. As has been shown, an individual may look pure and yet be a half-bred ... Yet one is homogeneous, the other heterogeneous in respect to almost every obvious character, and the breeding test alone reveals the secret.[6]

We now know, Mason continued, that Galton's law of heredity – half from each parent and a quarter from each grandparent – cannot be said to hold true, because it only recognizes the effects of dominant inheritance and does not take into account hidden, recessive inheritance. Breeders should at least grasp the meaning of Mendelism, even if it is no use to them right now. "At the same time," Mason added, "as the writer is aware from practical experience a few simple experiments made with animals or plants will do more to assist the realization of modern conceptions of heredity than all the books on the subject put together."[7]

The conviction that specialized breeding for purity more or less guaranteed consistency of type faltered after the Mendelian revolution. Evidently the occurrence of recessive features would not be winnowed out by breeding for what was perceived to promote homogeneity and through that process the deletion of inferior qualities. Charts and percentages (even if gathered from registry pedigrees) based only on the hereditary views of Galton would not be the answer. Under these conditions the idea that pedigrees guaranteed purity, a concept established in Bates's time, lost some of its credibility. The relationship of purity with quality correspondingly also became increasingly less tenable. Purity as an idea continued, though (as it always had), to carry much cultural cachet in terms of monetary worth. For that reason alone, specialization for purity did not go away. The idea that consistency of type could at least be encouraged by breeding for purity also endured, thereby reinforcing its value. While purity might not guarantee consistency of type, it was still believed to play some role in maintaining it. As a result, purity remained firmly fixed as one aspect of breeding even if a definition of it and its worth became ever more difficult and elusive. Which aspect of the purity concept – consistency of type or monetary value – in the end was more powerful (or more influential) historically speaking is hard to say, but the problem will be assessed more thoroughly in the third section of this book.

The theoretical work of the Mendelians might have fascinated practical breeders, but when the new geneticists started in the twentieth century to address more seriously first plant breeding and subsequently animal breeding from an improvement point of view, they often confronted practical breeders over method and general outlook. A particularly good example of practical breeder and scientist clash can be seen in the 1913 debate between scientist Raymond Pearl and practical breeder H.H. Stoddard over chicken breeding. American biologist Pearl, while working at the Maine Experiment Station between 1907 and 1916, was one of the few researchers interested in farm animal improvement, a situation which made him unusual. Pearl hoped his experiments would reveal how hereditary laws governing egg laying operated, and therefore what breeding strategies made the best sense for farmers.

Pearl concluded that practical breeders should avoid the "childishly simple scheme of breeding like to like." He stated that the method was counterproductive because it did not take into account (which his tests did) the importance of the male in egg-laying ability or capitalize on that fact.[8] Stoddard, a life-long chicken breeder and journalist, disagreed with Pearl's approach and theories. While Stoddard accepted the idea that males were important, he argued that experience proved females "had a great deal to say about" egg-laying capacity.[9] Furthermore, "like to like" breeding worked. The method might not result in consistently superior progeny, but it led to some offspring being as good as the parents "and some decidedly better," Stoddard wrote.[10] By breeding from the "decidedly better" progeny for the next generation, improvement was possible.

Pearl's comments could be unclear as to implication (an example being his assessment of relative male/female input to egg-laying ability), and as to actual breeding methodology (his emphasis on testing by quality of offspring and not on parentage was not evident in his publications), thereby undermining his arguments. It often remained difficult, even for scientists, to see how genetics could impact agricultural breeding of animals. For example, W.E. Castle (an American embryologist who turned to mammalian genetics after the rediscovery of Mendel's laws, and a professor at Harvard University) contended that, as far as animal breeding was concerned (especially the larger animals), traditional methods would continue to prevail for a considerable time. Farmers "breed animals as our fathers and grandfathers did because their time-honored methods succeed and we know of no reason for changing these methods," he wrote in a 1912 issue of the *American Breeders' Magazine*.[11]

Mendelism and Its Relationship to Animal Breeding: The Double-Cross Hybrid Breeding Method

A new turn of events began in 1917 when D.F. Jones (an American agricultural plant geneticist working at the Connecticut Experimental Research Station) started to focus on producing superior corn by using the geneticist experimental inbreeding and outcrossing method. For that method to work, however, it had to be made to overcome the problem of little or no improvement. Inbreeding reduced vigour, and while the crossing might return vigour to the plants or animals, it did not generate improvement over their original state before inbreeding had been practised on them. The stock simply returned to normal.

Jones hypothesized that a system involving multiple programs of inbreeding and outcrossing of inbred lines (later described as the double-cross hybrid method of breeding) could lead to improvement over the original stock.[12] He planned to produce a number of inbred and outcrossed lines of corn. He took two inbred lines and crossed them to produce a first-generation line. He took two other inbred lines and crossed them for another first-generation line. Next he took the two first-generation lines and crossed them to produce the final product, which was designed to show hybrid vigour, an evident jump in improvement. Jones postulated that he could, by the first cross of inbreds, restore the lines to the original fertility; and by the second cross, bring out superior improvement through hybrid vigour.[13] In order to maintain that level of hybrid vigour in corn over succeeding generations, seeds from the final cross would not be used for breeding. New generations demonstrating hybrid vigour would always be regenerated by stock belonging to the parent and grandparent generations. The method quickly attracted the attention of corn-breeding companies.

Corn companies were prepared to invest in experimenting with the new Jones method because they recognized it had the potential to generate guaranteed income. They could maintain economic viability by virtue of the fact that the producer would be a forced return customer. Collecting seeds for next year's planting would not result in similar corn, because hybridized plants and animals will not breed truly to their quality. The companies effectively would have a patent, which could be described as a biological lock. It would be some years, and after considerable effort and expense, however, before the method was more successful than traditional corn-breeding methods (which relied on selecting for lines that reproduced truly) at generating new seeds, in spite of propaganda suggesting otherwise.[14] Geneticists researching for the companies had achieved some success by the 1920s, enough to encourage farmers to begin buying double-cross hybrid seeds. This sort of breeding *volte face* would bring about a complete structural change to the American corn industry. As interest in breeding true lines collapsed, corn-producing farmers stopped breeding and collecting their own seeds for next year's crop. When the company-bred hybrid corn replaced farmer-bred corn, the industry became fractured in a way that was new to any agricultural industry: farmers were separated from both breeding and the management of breeding. The breeding arm of the industry fell under the control of corporate enterprise.

The managers of the corn companies believed the hybrid corn-breeding system could be successfully applied to chickens. They were willing to finance expensive experimental programs in order to find a way to achieve this end for the same reasons that they had invested in the method for corn breeding. Some corn companies, which already used professional geneticists, began hiring scientists to undertake poultry-breeding experiments, designed to produce what was known as "hybrid" chicks, namely birds that had been generated by some form of breeding involving hybridizing. The Wallace family, that is Henry A. Wallace, who developed the hybrid seed company Hi-Bred Corn Company in 1926 (renamed Pioneer Hi-Bred Corn Company in 1935), and his son Henry B. Wallace, initiated this effort to produce commercial hybrid chicks in 1936. By 1942 the Wallace family was selling hybrid egg-laying Leghorns under the name of Hy-Line.[15] (It is important to note that selection methods used to achieve these hybrid chicks were generally kept secret, even if inbreeding and outcrossing lay at the heart of the matter.) Farmers producing eggs soon no longer bred their own hens, but instead bought chicks from the corn companies breeding chickens. Genetics had entered the world of farm animal breeding when the new corporate approach took precedence.

Of primary significance to this transition was the fractured nature of the traditional chicken-breeding world in the 1930s within the United States, where the revolution began, a situation which ultimately divided the breeding arm from the producing arm of the industry. An escalating separation had been developing since the 1890s between breeders and chicken farmers keeping hens to produce eggs. A major underlying divisive factor in the chicken industry throughout this period related to the gender of people functioning within the two sectors: breeders were increasingly men only, while producers were overwhelmingly women. The breeders themselves encouraged a greater industry division than gendered labour would imply.

Many chicken breeders worked with inbreeding and crossing inbred lines, especially to promote beauty, and by following such strategies had tended for years to separate themselves from ordinary chicken farmers, who were women. North American chicken breeders themselves were also hopelessly divided in outlook by the 1920s, a situation which in the end created a sort of breeding vacuum. The adherence of the American Poultry Association to the Standard of Perfection, which was based on phenotype (or physical appearance), undermined attempts by some breeders to breed for utility. The resulting division in the breeding world also seemed to encourage a general loss of knowledge of the classic breeding methodology set out by such renowned poultry breeders as I.K. Felch and H.H. Stoddard. All of these factors fed into a situation which made it difficult for chicken farmers to breed birds themselves. The hatchery industry (comprised of commercial enterprises that bought eggs from breeders and incubated these to produce baby chicks) promoted this trend, and acted as another wedge between the breeding and producing arms of the chicken industry. Producers, separated from the process of breeding, began to demand hybrid stock when the companies made it available through hatcheries.[16] Successful American breeding companies joined similar ones that had arisen in Europe by the 1950s in dominating worldwide chicken breeding. The biological lock had been the primary corporate driver. Corporate enterprise stood to gain from this development and in fact made it happen. The transition brought with it a theoretical shift with respect to agricultural breeding: hybridizing, or inbreeding and outcrossing for offspring with hybrid vigour, would replace true breeding lines. The collapse of traditional approaches to breeding methods which emphasized the true line breeding of birds fed into the situation.[17]

The double-cross hybrid chicken method did not penetrate other animal-breeding industries to the same degree, but that fact did not result from lack of trying.[18] It had little effect, for example, on either dairy or beef breeding. Inherent characteristics of the "genetic" method of breeding and industry structure both played a role in deterring any such change. The cost of the individual animals and their slow reproduction made breeding by this method a difficult and lengthy process in cattle, and therefore discouraged the involvement of corporate enterprise. Tens of thousands of chickens had been required to find superior lines capable of leading to the terminal animal put out for sale, and, since cows produce one calf a year, it was difficult (and prohibitively costly) to generate similar numbers. Experiments on dairy cattle, however, commanded considerable attention from academic institutions. People in both Europe and the United States questioned if crossbreeding, and even inbreeding and crossing inbred lines, would improve the productivity of dairy cows. A number of crossbreeding or inbreeding experiments, designed to find answers, took place between 1906 and 1969. Results were inconclusive, providing little incentive for the dairy industry to abandon traditional methods.[19] (By 1980 it was evident that crossbreeding of Holsteins showed no improved production over pure Holsteins. They exceeded crossbreds for general performance by 10 per cent.)[20]

The structure of the dairy industry did not lend itself to the hybrid method either. Ordinary dairymen became part of the breeding arm in a way that was never true of ordinary chicken producers. While dairymen made their living from the milk their cows produced, they needed to breed those cows in order to generate that milk, a situation which would intimately connect them to the breeding world. Over the years dairymen worked ever more closely with breed and government organizations in most countries of the world, and supplied the data on milk yields that in turn drove their selection plans and those of the elite breeders. Purebred breeders and ordinary dairymen were also united by their focus on the production of true breeding lines. The increasing masculinization of the producing arm – milking had traditionally been women's work, while the breeding arm had tended to be male-dominated – reinforced this interconnected structure of the industry in a way that had not been true in the chicken situation.

Inbreeding and subsequent crossing techniques seemed at first glance to be amenable to beef breeding because of the role that crossing of breeds traditionally played in it. One successful Canadian chicken breeder, Don Shaver, undertook to introduce the hybrid corn-breeding method to the North American beef industry because of this longstanding interest in crossbreeding, and failed to do so.[21] The international organization of the breeding sector and of the industry generally explained why. The practical breeder arm of the beef industry comprised two distinct groups who functioned together: the purebred breeders, who created seed stock, and farmers (known as cow/calf operators), who kept cows to produce calves designed to be slaughtered for meat. Cow/calf farmers effectively multiplied animals designated for the meat industry, but they also acted independently as breeders themselves. Cow/calf farmers bought from purebred breeders, and used that stock to crossbreed in various ways in order to generate calves for the meat industry. Purebred breed associations, well established by this time, and government encouraged the reliance of cow/calf farmers on purebred bulls in their crossbreeding programs.

Final production involved what were known as "feeder" farmers, or feeders. The feeder farmers acquired the calves from the cow/calf farmers and fed the stock until it was ready for slaughter. The whole structure was tied together by the fact that the feeders decided what stock they wanted from the cow/calf operators, and the cow/calf operators decided what purebred cattle they would bring into their programs and how they would combine the genetics of those animals. From early times, cow/calf farmers had tried to utilize hybrid vigour by crossing bulls of a certain breed or type on cows with a different genetic background, but they resisted biological locks which hindered their control over breeding for feeder demand.[22] Since both breeder sectors and the final producing arm played a role in how breeding proceeded, the breeding and producing arms were strongly linked together, a situation which discouraged corporate involvement in breeding.

The Rise of Quantitative Genetics

Different strategies emanating out of genetics would direct dairy and beef breeding by the 1970s, strategies that were akin to practical breeding outlooks because of their affinity to tenets arising from force theory (namely true line breeding and generational change). These developments emerged after a major reorientation within the broad field of genetics had taken place. The 1920s had seen the rise of population genetics, which initiated a shift and widening in the focus of geneticists. Population genetics would view biometry (namely the study of changes within and across populations), as well as Mendelian experimental breeding, as being important to understanding the evolutionary process.[23] Neither faction, as a result, was considered antagonistic to Darwinism. Although the primary significance of biometry's contribution to population genetics related to this revaluation of Darwinism, the union of biometry with Mendelism would be highly significant for practical animal breeding. Effectively, ancient, practical animal-breeding concepts could now be introduced to the newly broadened field of genetics. The study of gradual change within populations over time was possible. Traits observed in animals – milk yields or egg-laying strength, for example – might be assessed quantitatively, meaning by degree of strength, across generations. Genetics was now in a position to make itself applicable to practical animal breeding outside the sophisticated systems of hybridizing.

It took Jay Lush, an American animal geneticist at Iowa State University, to see that population genetics offered new avenues for artificial selection strategies.[24] Lush intended to devise breeding plans which would modify true line breeding but would also fit with the existing structure of livestock industries. He wrote extensively about the historical background of livestock breeding within both contexts. Lush recognized that purebred breeding had emphasized individuals and that evaluation of type rested largely on phenotype (physical appearance) verified by the show ring.[25] While he saw the role of the show ring in breeding as a complicated issue, Lush admitted that at present there was no other way to identify good breeding animals of many species than by exhibition results.[26] He was most concerned with assessing the effects that inbreeding had on family groups or strains, and on the predictability of results from different breeding plans within that framework.[27] What selection strategies worked best? Did breeding half-siblings to each other, for example, bring better results than mating cousins?[28]

Lush drew on the views of two of the scientists concerned with evolution and credited with bringing about the rise of population genetics. Sewall Wright's theories concerning the effects of inbreeding proved highly significant to Lush.[29] R.A. Fisher's important 1918 paper, which argued that inheritance and change resulted from the interaction of many genes over time within populations (a theory known as the infinitesimal model), was equally critical, if not more so, to Lush's evolving ideas.[30] Over the 1930s and 1940s, Lush united the visions of Wright and Fisher and designed new systems to fine tune existing breeder practices.[31] In the process he removed Darwinism and its concern with evolution – so embedded in biometry, early Mendelism, and population genetics – from the practical problem of heredity under artificial selection.[32] Wright and Fisher might have played a role in the development of Lush's ideas; however, it was Lush himself who invented a deviation from population genetics, thereby creating quantitative genetics, also known also as animal genetics. In essence, quantitative genetics differed from population genetics in that it focused on alterations brought about by artificial selection, while population genetics addressed changes under natural selection. (Quantitative genetic principles, however, would be useful in various disciplines.) Lush believed by 1950 that quantitative genetics had started to influence animal breeding by moving it away from some of the tenets, namely emphasis on the individual, basic to the purebred system. He argued that "the quantizing of breeding plans [was] beginning to replace fairy tales and wishful thinking."[33]

Important to quantitative genetics from the beginning were better statistics to evaluate strategies used in artificial selection. As early as 1913, American statistician G.W. Snedecor at Iowa State University began devising statistics specifically for use in agriculture.[34] (Pearson and Fisher had been interested in applying statistics to the biological problems of evolution and human progress – namely the results of natural selection, not artificial selection.) Lush was important to the development of agricultural statistics, particularly those designed by his student L.N. Hazel, and Hazel's student C.R. Henderson. Henderson became interested in improving methods for properly identifying superior breeding bulls. It had become clear that a bull's value varied under different environmental conditions (feed levels and weather, for example). Henderson wanted to develop a statistical way of neutralizing these effects in order to provide an unbiased assessment of breeding bulls. In the end he invented BLUP (best linear unbiased prediction), which overcame the difficulties of unequal conditions affecting bulls.[35]

Quantitative Genetics and Cattle Breeding

On the basis of Lush's theories and evolving statistics as early as the 1940s, scientists turned their attention to livestock industries which supported both purebred and true line breeding, most specifically dairy cattle. They worked with (and needed) the data collected by dairymen who kept records of their cows' milk output, hoping to make that data yield clearer information on the relative value of sires. A British population geneticist from the University of Cambridge, Alan Robertson, was particularly significant in efforts to improve dairy cows by focusing statistics on the location of bulls that produced better daughters. Robertson studied principles of quantitative genetics under both Lush and Wright in the United States, before starting research at the Animal Unit Research Centre at Edinburgh after the Second World War.[36] The advent of artificial insemination (AI), and by the 1950s the ability to freeze semen, allowed him to be more effective in statistically testing males for the production of good daughters.[37] With the aid of international organizations like Interbull (founded in Sweden in the 1980s, and which collected data on milking cows from around the world) as well as the use of computers, quantitative genetics revolutionized dairy cattle breeding on a worldwide scale.[38] Emphasis on statistical quantification and its use to test males for their ability to produce good daughters evidently did not place a gene architecture approach at the centre of livestock genetics. The genetic makeup of a bull was both unknown and considered non-essential for finding good results. Clearly the force theory described this selection approach better than did gene architecture theory. The specific focus on bulls was also reminiscent of one of Bakewell's most noteworthy force theory principles, namely emphasis on the progeny test through the production of males because of that sex's ability to generate more data.

It helped that the international dairy industry's structure (namely the integral role of the ordinary dairy farmer in breeding good milking cows) was amenable to principles arising from the new animal science. The dairy associations were prepared to work with government and information arising from genetics. The North American purebred dairy associations had in fact initiated data collection before the advent of genetics itself.[39] From the beginning, breed associations agreed to cooperate with academic institutions.[40] In doing so, breed associations moved from the emphasis in purebred breeding on ancestry breeding (reliance on parental or earlier background) to Bakewell's view that the excellence of an animal, from a breeding perspective, should be based on the quality of its offspring, namely on the basis of the progeny test.

Quantitative genetics did not penetrate beef breeding either as easily or as early as it did dairy breeding. Industry structure was one problem. The beef industry did not lend itself to generating adequate data. The beef industry (large herds with minimal management) discouraged the extensive use of AI, and that fact alone hindered statistical genetic work in beef cattle: the data needed did not exist. (As of 2003, less than 5 per cent of the world's beef cattle were artificially inseminated.)[41] The attitude of the purebred beef associations was another problematic issue. These associations resisted change. It was primarily the fact that the Thoroughbred horse culture was so strongly embedded within the purebred beef industry that inflamed geneticists throughout this period.[42] Attitudes of American organizations serve as an example of international patterns. The purebred beef cattle associations in the United States, in control of any genetic advancement from their beginnings in the 1880s, continued until into the 1960s to evaluate breeding worth on the basis of ancestry, show ring success, and subjective visual appraisal. The influence of purebred animals, designed within that framework, could be felt throughout the industry. The terminal crossbreds that comprised the end beef product were generated by combinations of purebred cattle whose breeding had been regulated by the breed associations.

The first association effort to provide a more objective view of purebred quality (and therefore useable data for eventually testing the quality of the progeny in order to assess the worth of the parents, most notably sires) was the Red Angus Association, which in 1959 required weaning weights to be provided before pedigree registration was possible. Over the 1960s other beef breed associations developed performance-recording programs, although the Angus association remained the only one that required data reporting. It was largely the demands of American feeder operators in the 1940s and 1950s that led to improvements in recording the performance of purebred beef cattle. A move to better orchestrate improvement programs began in 1965 and resulted in the Beef Improvement Federation, formed in 1967. The breed associations maintained a strong voice in that organization.[43]

In the 1970s the purebred associations, particularly those supporting the newly imported European breeds, began to adopt performance evaluation systems based on a BLUP design. Evaluation systems revolved around what was known as EPD (estimated progeny difference) for a variety of traits. An EPD is a prediction of an animal's likelihood of passing on a trait in relation to breed average for that trait. While the most common EPDs calculated were for birth weight, weaning weight, and yearling weight as gain per day after birth, the number of EPDs expanded over the years in relation to the capacity of computers to handle complicated statistics. The gradual adoption of EPDs as breeding strategies resulted in a beef cattle revolution. These changes helped defuse antagonism between scientist and purebred breeder.

The beef cattle revolution of the 1970s reflected, not just an increased use of statistical principles, but also the importation of new beef breeds to replace herds ruined by excessive reverence to show ring style.[44] By the late 1950s the overpowering emphasis over many decades on the short blocky type (relentlessly selected for by judges in spite of emerging evidence from feeders, if not agricultural colleges, that stock improvement was not promoted by the type)[45] had led to inferior animals in the Hereford, Angus, and Shorthorn breeds. Feeder farmers and meat consumers increasingly did not find stock from those breeds acceptable.[46] Feeder farmers found the cattle expensive to raise relative to slaughter values, while consumers ended up with meat having a high ratio of fat or waste. Avoidance of the three breeds that had apparently been ruined by show ring dynamics led to the importation of animals (Charolais and Simmentals, for example) which were larger and leaner. By 2000 the old Hereford and Angus breeds had recovered in importance within the new purebred beef industry structure. They managed to do so by adopting standards that reflected more useful cattle as to size and frame (which matched that of the Continental breeds), and also through the impact of quantitative genetics. The Shorthorn breed made efforts to change phenotypic style (physical appearance) through breeding but did not recover its earlier prestige or its dominance within the industry. (The beef cattle revolution of the 1970s and its effect on the affairs of certain breeds will be elaborated on in more detail later in this book, specifically in parts of chapters 3, 7, and 8.)

Thoroughbred Horse Breeding in the Age of Mendelism and Quantitative Genetics

Developments in both Mendelian and quantitative genetics affected how purebred breeding operated, especially in relation to attitudes towards the meaning of purity and to ancestry-based selection. A gradual shift back to the Bakewellian roots behind purebred breeding took place. At the heart of the matter was the changing role that pedigrees played in breeding methodology and views on how heredity worked. Happenings in the world of Thoroughbred horse breeding, that other arm that comprised purebred breeding and the one which had brought public recording of pedigrees into the purebred system, show a sharp contrast to the shifts seen in the purebred breeding of dairy and beef cattle.

Horse breeders clung to the culture of their past, evidenced by their adoption of statistics to work with pedigree, ancestry-driven breeding, rather than with statistical progeny testing, or the concept that heredity should be assessed in terms of groups or populations. The horse breeders elaborated and developed different theories that rested on eighteenth-century ancestry breeding, individual worth, and pedigrees which supported the value of both. Such strategies revealed a continuing affinity to Galton's ancestral law, thereby indicating an allegiance to beliefs that predated the birth of genetics. Two examples, which are still part of Thoroughbred horse breeding culture today, suffice to demonstrate this pattern: the use of dosage theory and the figure system.

Dosage theory originated from the work of a Frenchman, J.J. Vuillier, in 1902. He examined the pedigrees of successful race horses to the twelfth generation and noted that there were similarities in that fifteen stallions and one mare appeared in all of them with roughly the same frequency. He devised a sort of formula or recipe for creating the ideal race horse. If one selected a horse that lacked the relative "dosage" needed to recreate a needed pedigree, the animal mated to that horse should compensate for that deficiency through his/her pedigree. Vuillier drew heavily on Francis Galton's interviews with Thoroughbred horse breeders. A foal represented a blend of hereditary material, usually thought of as being "blood," a conception that fitted with force manipulation thinking. "Blood" meant that some unknown laws existed driving the way inheritance worked, even if they were not understood. Dosage theory attracted attention throughout the period when animal genetics developed over the twentieth century. The third Aga Khan relied heavily on dosage during the 1930s when breeding Thoroughbreds. Vuillier's work also influenced Italian Franco Varola, who wrote about breeding in the 1970s, and modified dosage theory. Further modifications would emerge in the 1980s and 1990s. Dosage remained concerned only with analysis of superior horses within the male line, and still influences Thoroughbred breeding decisions today.[47]

The figure system is based on the work of nineteenth-century Australian Bruce Lowe, who spent years tracing every mare appearing in the General Stud Book back to her "taproot" in the original edition. He then gave numbers to each of these families, ranging from 1 to 43, and related mares to male winners of the great races over time. His work was carried on in the twentieth century, even though DNA testing showed that the pedigrees on which the figure system was based were often flawed. That situation did not deter breeders from using statistics arising from the figure system in making breeding decisions. Pedigrees were at the heart of the figure system, as was reliance on ancestry breeding and emphasis on individuals. It seemed evident to geneticists that the methods used to breed race horses had not improved their speed in the last half-century before 2014.[48] The lack of AI use – not allowed for registration in the Jockey Stud Book – did not help matters. With enforced natural service in place, stallion owners dictate stud fees and keep them high. But the restriction on AI use means that insufficient data exists on breeding males for quantifying the relative quality of stallions against each other. Stallion owners control much of the way Thoroughbred horse breeding proceeds, because they play a critical role in directing how effective progeny testing will be with respect to males.

Quantitative Genetics and Biomathematics

Quantitative genetics introduced principles reminiscent of Bakewell's to both purebred dairy and beef cattle breeding, and at the same time initiated a shift away from Thoroughbred horse breeding culture. While many quantitative genetic principles in fact simply pushed purebred breeding back to its Bakewellian roots, that situation was not obvious to breeders. They did not see the new emphasis on progeny testing and quantification (over ancestry breeding and individual worth), or the subsequent reliance on statistics, as being a reintroduction of strategies that had originated in eighteenth-century Bakewellianism. Breeders viewed these changes as emanating out of the science of genetics. The vastly superior statistics used for quantification in the twentieth century, when compared to the tools available in the eighteenth, helped make the techniques look completely innovative. AI and its power to progeny test more effectively completely changed the landscape, and thereby also helped to hide Bakewellian foundations. Because the shifts meshed well with the breeding arm's traditional framework, a revolution was possible without reshaping the general industry, another factor in masking the foundations of the past. Basic historic industry structure remained the same: breeder and producer were linked together through the production and use of true breeding lines, and breed associations continued to have relevance by virtue of the fact that they collected the data used in quantitative analysis.

Changes in cattle breeding clearly showed that quantitative (or statistical) genetics provided effective strategies to improve animals, and as a result, modified the methodology of the hybrid chicken breeders. While the companies maintained their faith in inbreeding and crossing, by the 1960s they used strain crosses from parental lines with low levels of inbreeding (which had undergone selection using quantitative genetics), thereby abandoning the emphasis on extreme inbreeding for the lines used to make the hybrid cross.[49] Everywhere in animal breeding circles, the main contribution of genetics seemed to rest primarily on mathematics. It was a situation that many geneticists were aware of and increasingly concerned about. While studying biological issues in terms of statistics had been practised since the time of Bakewell, advances in biomathematics and statistics under quantitative genetics presented some scientists with important questions. How could it be argued, for example, that assessing biological functions with no knowledge of the dynamics that caused them made sense? Ultimately what was mathematics and what was biology? At what point, in other words, did a biomathematical study cease to be one of biology and become one simply of mathematics?[50] Heavy emphasis on statistics in aspects of genetic research, particularly relevant when viewing quantitative genetics, appeared to these geneticists to be taking science too far from its main purpose, namely understanding gene dynamics. Advances in molecular genetics by the 1970s intensified that sense, helping to make quantitative genetics lose some of its aura. The next chapter addresses the subject of molecular genetics, as well as genomics, in animal breeding. We will see if the approach of quantitative genetics would be completely superseded.

Chapter Three

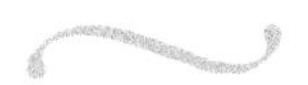

Animal Breeding in the Age of Molecular Genetics, Genomics, and Epigenetics, 1990–2020

Molecular genetics (initiated in the late 1940s, but further stimulated by the discovery of DNA's structure in 1953) attracted increasing attention over the period of quantitative genetics' growth. The 1970s, however, brought the really dramatic breakthroughs which threatened to change the entire landscape as far as attitudes to statistics and quantitative genetics were concerned. Recombinant DNA technology, which allowed for the transferring of sections of DNA from one organism into another, made it possible to study the functioning of actual genes at the molecular level.[1] The sense that gene interaction could be understood tended to bring the gene architecture approach back to the forefront of research and concurrently to push quantitative genetics, with its emphasis on statistics, into the background. A transition period for animal breeding appeared to be imminent. Geneticists began to ask, as well: Could or would molecular genetics replace quantitative genetics in animal breeding? When scientists who used quantitative genetic tactics (animal biologists, evolutionary biologists, population geneticists, agricultural geneticists, and statisticians, to name a few) gathered together in 1976 at Ames, Iowa for their first international conference, this question, the nature of quantitative genetics itself, and its approach to studies in genetics stimulated much discussion.

O. Kempthorne, a statistician and geneticist from Iowa State University, began the meetings by defining what quantitative genetics meant, and in the process tried to put to rest "the not-uncommon tendency to regard a conference on quantitative genetics as a conference on population genetics." He continued with the following statements, which clearly defined quantitative genetics and set the discipline within its historic context.

> We wished to organize a conference, then, in quantitative genetics and not in population genetics as it is conventionally understood ... Many of the

> ideas of conventional population genetics are important to quantitative genetics. And, contrariwise, it seems clear that many of the ideas of conventional quantitative genetics are relevant to population genetics … Part of the distinction between the two areas is simply that quantitative genetics should be called experimental population genetics, with the emphasis on the word "experimental", connoting that we make genetic populations by controlled operations, while conventional population genetics is primarily observational population genetics, trying to understand populations that have arisen by natural and not humanly directed processes … The big thrust [of quantitative genetics] has been towards the species of direct relevance to the food needs of the human species, and this explains why quantitative genetics is dominated by [those interested in] animal and plant breed[ing].[2]

But, he admitted, quantitative genetics had not been able to understand the genetic architecture of traits in agricultural plants and animals that were economically valuable, a serious shortcoming within the contemporary environment of genetics.[3] R.E. Comstock, an agricultural plant geneticist in the United States, concurred, believing the discipline was inadequate in many ways, in spite of the fact that it had offered major contributions to breeding designs. "There are significant issues in the realm of quantitative genetics that have not been resolved," he stated. "Some of these appear tractable, others relatively intractable … It appears from the perspective of the breeder that quantitative genetics still has a challenging future."[4] D.L. Harris, an American livestock geneticist, pointed out the significance of historical breeding. "It is well to remember," Harris noted, "that animal breeding was a serious activity of many stockmen prior to the discovery of [the] Mendelian basis of inheritance."[5] He implied value in practical thinking: early breeders had managed to breed without sophisticated statistics or Mendelism.

For R.C. Lewontin, that was not the point. An American evolutionary biologist and population geneticist at Harvard University, Lewontin believed in the application of techniques from molecular biology to questions of genetic variation and evolution, and would pioneer strategies to do so throughout his life. He used the black box metaphor to explain why avoidance of molecular genetics did not serve any branch of genetics well. When causes can be attributed to bringing about certain results but the laws governing how the results come about remain unknown, this is a "black box" way of looking at a problem.[6] The dynamics between cause and result are hidden or encased in a black box. In effect, Lewontin equated black box thinking with biometric thinking. Since he believed the black box approach had no place in science, as far as he was concerned, neither did the attitude of quantitative genetics. In effect, Lewontin reintroduced the conflict that had plagued naturalists before the rise of genetics and subsequently scientists before the rise of population genetics. Did cell theory (gene architecture theory) or force theory (black box theory) serve artificial selection breeding methods best?

Lewontin elaborated on his point of view. Quantitative genetics may be used to predict results of certain selection methods through statistics, he stated, but we know nothing about the genetic architecture which would dictate the effectiveness of any such method. Genes and gene interaction "were treated as if occurring inside a black box" only knowable through observable output. In effect, quantitative genetics constituted "an attempt to produce knowledge by a systemization of ignorance."[7] He went on: "We need to know the relations between gene and organism, how gene action … is translated into phenotype. The knowledge about these questions can come to us only by opening up the black box whose outer shape we have so far been describing, and seeing what the machinery inside really looks like."[8] We should look to the methods used and the work done by molecular geneticists, Lewontin noted, adding, "Our models of quantitative genetics must either take cognizance of these findings or else show how they are, in fact, irrelevant because of the robustness of our theory."[9]

A reviewer of the 1976 conference addressed the statistical stance embedded in quantitative genetics in relation to the approach of molecular genetics somewhat differently:

> In recent years, the once thriving field of quantitative genetics (QG) has fallen on hard times. Both the discipline and its practitioners have been criticized for a total failure to deal with the genetic … underpinning [of] the phenotype. Such attacks are more than a little unfair … Quantitative genetics is nothing more (and nothing less) than a convenient statistical construct whose prime function is to permit estimation and testing of a set of summary measures … Since nary a gene is seen, the fact that these summary measures convey any genetic information at all must be viewed as a splendid accomplishment. It is precisely for the analysis of those phenotypes which are hopelessly complex that quantitative genetics was designed.[10]

Lewontin might argue that molecular genetics was the way to go for animal breeding strategies, but in 1976 that simply was still not possible, in spite of the rise of recombinant DNA technology. He and reviewers of the 1976 conference had also been somewhat unfair in claiming that quantitative geneticists took no interest in, or ignored the potential of, molecular genetics for practical animal breeding. Well before the rise of recombinant DNA technology, Alan Robertson had stated at the Genetics Commission of the European Association of Animal Production, meeting in 1969 in Helsinki, that quantitative geneticists should be paying more attention to information arising from molecular genetics.[11] He himself had tried to find a way to develop artificial selection strategies on the basis of DNA as early as 1961 by looking at blood groups found in highly producing dairy cows. Prior to 1980, the only suitable way to look for specific molecular structures was to assess blood groups. Blood groups, however, had no visible effect on any traits of interest. Evidently, using blood groups to find traits of interest, molecularly speaking, in animal populations would not work. The situation had not really changed by 1976 when geneticists met for the conference. There still was no way to use molecular genetics in selection methods based on quantifying the strength of trait inheritance.

Nor did molecular technology appear over the 1980s to help them develop any usable strategy. As a result, at the second quantitative conference held in 1987, it was apparent that statistical studies (effectively black box thinking or force theory) persisted in dominating quantitative genetics. Quantitative geneticists might be quite prepared to incorporate a more molecular outlook if it worked with the idea of statistical change over generations and across populations, but the reality was that by the late 1980s the theoretical approach was still far ahead of technology that could put it into practice. Molecular genetics and technology would soon, however, suggest exciting, innovative ways to develop strategies for breeding animals. Changes were on the horizon, and the fate of quantitative genetics would hang in the balance.

Molecular Genetics and Animal Breeding: Marker and Microsatellite Technology

The gene architecture approach supported the idea that finding an isolated gene which acted as a marker, or a DNA sequence (stretch of DNA) responsible for the inheritance of economically important traits, would be invaluable for making breeding decisions.[12] By the 1990s a new technology, which looked at microsatellites (that is, repeat stretches in DNA which could be seen in relation to genes believed to affect quantitative traits), made that seem possible.[13] Mapping markers might provide a way to make selection factors rest on DNA profiles. Even single markers could be touted as important when it came to breeding selection, but it continued to be unclear how useful any form of marker technology was for breeding purposes and whether the expense of DNA testing of animals made economic sense.

The role of corporate enterprise in establishing and selling marker technology further muddied the water, as can be seen in the case of beef tenderness markers. In the early 1990s, two markers for marbling and beef tenderness were located in cattle from experiments done on the DNA of beef Shorthorns in Australia.[14] After 2000, three companies started to promote the markers by offering genetic testing for them, and North American Shorthorn breeders in particular were targeted for sales. Favourable results could be useful to breeders, the companies argued, especially when it became evident that carriers of the markers were not particularly common. Shorthorn breeder interest in the test was relatively short lived, in keeping with the general practical view that too much focus on single factors was not likely to increase the strength of any valuable trait. A few breeders used the test as a marketing device, but by about 2006 even that focus had gone into decline. There was little evidence that the markers actually proved anything in relation to breeding for economic traits, as later studies would point out. In 2007 an independent scientific study was done to see how viable the companies' claims were that genetic testing of this nature was worthwhile. The conclusion was that the tests might result in a higher percentage of choice carcasses, but "independent, third-party validation of commercial DNA tests [would] provide some assurance to producers that DNA-based tests perform in accordance with the claims of the marketing companies and [might] help to generate some of the data required to facilitate the integration of marker data into the national cattle evaluation."[15]

Microsatellite technology might not work well for locating inheritable economic traits, but it could be used to find markers locating the DNA responsible for recessive defects. The ability to find carriers (namely animals with one recessive copy for the defect and a dominant copy against it) meant that they could be removed from breeding herds, thereby reducing the incidence of defective animals (who carried two recessive copies) being born. The development of technology to locate such carriers mushroomed in the early twenty-first century. Breeders, however, did not always use the technology to reduce the incidence of defective progeny. An example of this pattern could be seen in the reactions of North American Shorthorn breeders to a test for the defect Tibial Hemimelia, known as TH. The Shorthorn story in relation to defect markers (that is, the location of carrier animals having only one copy for TH) elucidates the fact that simply having the technology to change the course of breeding is not enough to make that happen.

The position of a breed in its general industry, in conjunction with its historical breeding culture, created powerful factors in driving how new technologies would be used in actual breeding programs. The declining influence of Shorthorns in the North American beef world at the end of the twentieth century was behind the problem. Shorthorns had not recovered in popularity with cow/calf operators or feeder farmers (even for crossbreeding purposes) after the quantitative genetic and importation revolution of the 1970s. As Shorthorn numbers fell in relation to the growth in other breeds, it became difficult to incorporate quantitative genetics (with its reliance on data collection) effectively into Shorthorn breeding operations, thereby encouraging the dominance of the purebred method alone (with its interconnected base of pedigree keeping, ancestry and individual worth, and the importance of the show system). In many ways the role of the show ring in Shorthorn affairs by 2000 was reminiscent of Lush's views about its power over breeding in the 1930s. Since marketing via showing is fundamental to purebred breeding, Shorthorn breeders logically remained concerned with show markets. The show market, however, became so important to this breed that the continuation of genetic defects could be seen almost as a positive good. A vicious circle developed. More show breeding meant less utility breeding, and less utility breeding meant a smaller commercial market, which in turn drove more interest in show breeding.

TH defective calves (unable to live, with shortened to non-existent hind legs and often the brain cavity open) had begun to appear in the 1990s as a result of inbreeding to certain desired sire lines for show purposes. There was some sense that the defect was simply covered up, perhaps because affected individuals emanated out of valuable exhibition individuals. By 1999 the problem had been labelled as TH.[16] In 2002 Jon Beever (a molecular geneticist at the University of Illinois) detected the recessive defect in DNA, which resulted from a one-third deletion of gene *ALX4*. He, with the collaboration of geneticist David Steffen of the University of Nebraska-Lincoln, developed a test using microsatellite technology, which located carriers by revealing they had one copy for deletion in the gene.[17]

Because THC (TH carriers or "dirty") animals were valuable to breeders, they became increasingly reluctant to drop THC breeding lines, as the wording of sale catalogues between 2006 (when a test for TH carriers was available) and 2016 makes clear. In the 2006 fall sales, breeders announced that all entries were THF (TH free or "clean") unless otherwise stated, with THC stock being listed.[18] But as early as 2007, subtle changes could be found in the wording of the catalogues. TH tests were stated as "pending."[19] The trend away from noting carriers in catalogues, and instead relying on the "pending" label, became increasingly common after 2007. Some catalogues made no mention of even "pending" TH status, while known THC bulls and cows were the parents of calves offered in the sale.[20] Sales were based on the fact that THC cattle won at shows. Uniformity of judges' decisions had set a trend for style accepted in the show ring, and breeders favoured breeding to that type by whatever means it took because the primary market for Shorthorns, many believed, was for show cattle. As one person stated on the Internet chat room known as *Steerplanet*, "You cannot win with free [THF] genetics ... I know it hurts like hell but it is the truth. YOU CANNOT WIN WITH CLEAN GENETICS."[21] Even geneticists tended to accept the conviction that THC animals had a propensity to demonstrate characteristics favoured by judges.[22] The desire for show ring success and the conviction that the TH factor helped create successful show stock could even bring breeders to purposely breed THC carriers with each other. Perhaps the perceived benefits bestowed by carrying one copy of the gene would somehow be magnified and not end up with a defective calf.[23]

Breeders argued that markets (in this case for show cattle) should drive pedigree status. "Let the cream rise regardless [of] who breeds it," reasoned another, who was answered with, "That's exactly right. And if someone wants to breed carriers, then let them. The buyers will determine if there is a market or not."[24] THC cattle sell because they win at shows; the market wants THC cattle, therefore they should be pedigreed. Attitudes of this nature made it impossible for the American Shorthorn Association to act more aggressively. (Canadian breeders were generally more receptive to the idea of restrictions regarding TH, but their close working relationship with American breeders and their use of popular American breeding lines precluded any concerted effort to disallow registration of THC animals.) It is interesting to note, in contrast, the way British breeders and their association handled the TH issue. The Beef Shorthorn Society of Britain required testing for TH, and after early 2008 refused to allow entry of THC animals into Coates's Herd Book.[25]

Advanced microsatellite technology had clearly done little to change animal breeding methods by the end of the twentieth century. Work on DNA markers for increased production had been disappointing. In 1998 it was noted that "knowledge of genetic architecture [was] ... very limited for economic traits of farm animals."[26] Locating animals carrying the defect via microsatellite technology had not always been particularly effective in the reduction of defective animals. Both the finding of markers for economic traits and the use of markers to locate genetic defects in breeding programs seemed to be at a dead end. Molecular genetics, with its DNA-oriented approaches to breeding, had also failed to modify the dynamics of quantitative genetics with its statistical population outlook based on black box thinking (or force theory).

Genomics, Epigenetics, and Breeding

The rise of genomic research, which occurred while work on marker identification was going on, would ultimately preserve the black box (or force theory) outlook which lay behind quantitative genetics and bring that approach back to the forefront. Genomics, the study of DNA at the molecular level but across all chromosomes in any given species (as opposed to small sections or specific genes under recombinant DNA technology), had originally brought hope that the repeated failures to advance any real way of using DNA markers or even successfully locate such markers would be overcome.[27] The desire to understand the genetic architecture of traits inherited in a quantitative way finally seemed possible with the sequencing of animal genomes.[28] That, however, would not be the case.

It soon became evident that genomic technology, which located many thousands of random SNPs (single nucleotide polymorphisms), parts of so-called junk DNA and not protein-coding genes, did not enhance useful knowledge of the functioning of DNA for traits quantitatively and therefore did not endorse a gene architecture outlook. SNP technology supported the black box (or force theory) outlook of quantitative genetics. Certain SNP patterns, it became apparent, characterized bulls known through quantitative genetics to be superior.[29] That situation made them valuable in developing a test to assess superiority in bulls (particularly young ones) that had not been tested statistically under quantitative genetic principles. It could be assumed that animals with the same SNP profile as known good bulls, but with no data, were also superior. It was hard for some, though, to imagine that the sophisticated progeny testing of bulls over the past fifty years under quantitative genetics could be replaced with genomic testing. *Hoard's Dairyman* told breeders in 2008 that "Genome-tested bulls [might] soon be on the market," but we have no idea how genomic predictions will work out or whether they can and should replace the old progeny testing system.[30]

Genomic selection via SNPs also clearly negated the idea behind single trait marker theory, and instead favoured the infinitesimal model of R.A. Fisher, which argued that a large number of unknown genes (or even parts of the DNA that were not genes), acting with each other also in an unknown way, are responsible for a trait.[31] Geneticists were quick to point out this fundamental linkage to black box thinking, and its deviation away from gene architecture theory. In 2007 livestock geneticist J. van der Werf wrote that "this [SNP] approach seems to revert back to the black box, where the emphasis is on predicting generic variability for observed traits, rather than on understanding the underlying biology." He elaborated:

> Animal breeders have always been working with the "black box" containing the biology of the animal. They have had enormous impacts on the black box, but are only really aware of the outputs. Some animal breeding scientists have argued that understanding the black box is important, especially for understanding the relationship between productivity and fitness ... With the advent of molecular genetics, there seemed a new chance to embrace biology ... Yet, the hunt for quantitative trait loci has been relentless, while the application in breeding programmes is still rather disappointing, and the biology possibly becoming more complicated rather than clarified.[32]

If SNP technology was to work, it needed the input of data generated by quantitative genetics and purebred breeding, both of which offered information, statistically speaking.[33] Those adhering to the older inbreeding and subsequent crossing inbred lines method (that is, the chicken breeders) could not capitalize on such testing because breeding for terminal crosses (in terms of breeding potential) did not generate the necessary data. The fact that breeding companies kept their strains or lines secret, in order to protect intellectual property, did not help the situation. It was the international dairy industry that could provide the data needed to formulate a SNP test which could identify superior animals. The dairy industry had created a massive statistical base which rested on the work of quantitative geneticists, and even earlier of purebred breeders and ordinary dairymen. In 2008 a high-density panel, containing over fifty thousand SNP markers across the genome (known as the Bovine SNP50 BeadChip), was developed by the company Illumina in California. Illumina created the panel by comparing statistics that had identified the superior ability of three thousand bulls to produce good milking daughters with characteristics of their DNA profile.[34] When the BeadChip became available the following year, it proved to be highly accurate in locating quality dairy bulls, in spite of some earlier scepticism evident in dairy journals. (When the beef breeds collected genomic data on the basis of the BeadChip a few years later, they had to pool their genomic and quantitative genetic information together in order to generate adequate accuracy rates.)

It was soon clear, though, that the larger number of animals used to develop a test and the greater volume of SNPs profiled, the higher the accuracy rate. By assessing the genome in a more comprehensive fashion, in order to bring in a huge number of SNPs, it was possible to make better estimates of an individual's breeding worth. Complexity, Fisher's infinitesimal model theory, and black box or force theory thinking all took precedence over a genetic architecture approach in genomic methods of breeding.[35] In 2013, sixty years after the discovery of the molecular structure of DNA, *Nature* commented on the general elusiveness of understanding genetic architecture. "When the structure of DNA was first deduced, it seemed to supply the final part of a beautiful puzzle, the solution of which began with Charles Darwin and Gregor Mendel. The simplicity of that picture has proved too alluring."[36]

Genetics' interface with animal breeding has become more complicated after these dramatic genomic breakthroughs. Postgenomics, that is the period after roughly 2010 (or even beginning in 2007 with the completion of ENCODE, which mapped critical repeat selections of DNA), would be dominated by the theory of epigenetics, a term invented in the 1940s by Conrad Waddington, a British developmental biologist, geneticist, and philosopher. Waddington believed that phenotype (physical appearance) and genotype (genetic makeup) resulted from outside causes (possibly environmental) interacting with genes. As a result, the epigenetic theory held that the study of inheritance should see some modifications of phenotypic and genotypic expression as being beyond the interaction of genetic material in the DNA.[37] The theory re-emerged with force in the postgenomic era because genomics had made it clear that unknown factors, called "missing heritability," operated with the parts of DNA identified as defining a trait. The dynamics of the genome had proved to be far more complex than anyone had realized, and epigenetics presented a theoretical way out of the heritability mystery by suggesting that a holistic, all-embracing attitude to heredity should take precedence over genetic determinist approaches. Such an outlook, on the surface, fitted well with the vision of practical breeders. The attitude also harboured a Lamarckian view, namely that the environment could influence patterns of heredity. This approach, which had directed animal breeding from the time of Rome until the seventeenth century, had never really vanished from practical animal breeding theory.

Existing technology in the postgenomic era adds to the complexity of the picture. CRISPR Cas 9, for example, has the capacity to work with either inbreeding and outcrossing inbred lines for terminal crosses or breeding for true lines. The technology can alter the entire structure of DNA and therefore might be able to redesign the basic DNA of farm animals (many think it will).[38] (SNP technology only identifies the structure of existing DNA; CRISPR Cas 9 allows for its manipulation.) Whether CRISPR Cas 9 does so within a framework which supports hybridizing or aligns itself with true breeding lines remains to be seen. As in the case of SNP technology (and the tests that combine it with paternity, genetic defect carriers, and certain markers), corporate investment might fund the creation of a platform which breeders would buy and use in true line breeding. Who provides the input as to how to design a new DNA structure, however, is another interesting question. Corporate enterprise would not, under these conditions, necessarily take over breeding itself.

~

A pervasive division (even oscillation) between cell or gene architecture and force theoretical approaches on how to study heredity characterized geneticist theory, just as had been the case with naturalists over the nineteenth century. No such oscillation with respect to hereditary theory took place in the animal breeding world: the outlook, generally speaking, continued to rest, as it always had, on a general force theory which supported a black box view. A mutual approach to heredity (namely generalized black box attitudes) facilitated a genetic infiltration of science into practical breeding. The interface between genetics and practical animal breeding within the cattle industries, for example, was successful because the two groups held similar opinions concerning breeding theory. Both worked with the idea of breeding over generations for true lines to advance changes that were, in effect, quantitative. Their views varied only in that, before the 1940s and in keeping with purebred breeding, breeders had focused on individuals within such a framework, while quantitative geneticists (reminiscent of Bakewell) assessed such shifts on a population basis. The move by breeders to supporting quantitative changes as a population issue did not interfere with the historic structure of the industries. Quantitative genetics, then, fitted with general practical breeding theory and also industry structure. That was not the case with hybridizing or specific DNA studies. Only in the chicken industry did the hybridizing method revolutionize breeding, but it did so because the declining emphasis on true breeding lines and the subsequent separation of breeder from producer both helped to create an atmosphere conducive to such a method. Genomics has done little to change that underlying situation. Its greatest effects on breeding have been in relation to true breeding lines, and in many ways it is arguable that genomic technology (like SNP testing) is merely a molecular-genetic extension of quantitative genetics. The success of genomic breeding could only happen in conjunction with quantitative genetics. It remains to be seen how future technology and future breeding theory will fit into this picture.

Breeding methodology is the foundation of how we use animals. It underlies all aspects of our relationship to domestic animals. It has been seen here as a story, therefore, in its own right. The aims of breeding, meaning what to breed for, play a significant role in how we use animals, even if attitudes to what selection should be directed at have to work with breeding methodology. The next section looks at how different aims can orchestrate changes in animals and at the same time reflect aspects of human society.

SECTION TWO

What to Breed For: The Many Aims of Selection

Chapter Four

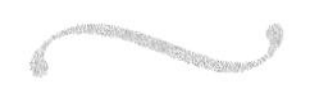

Specialization for Purpose and Animal Breeding

The wish to change animals results from breeding with certain objectives in mind. As a concept, therefore, the aims of selection differ from ideology behind method and are not driven by information arising from practical breeding or science. Selection aims employ any existing methods, proven through experience to alter phenotype, and can utilize science to achieve ends. They often involve the state (through support structures which encourage certain moves to specific aspects of improvement) and drive organizational structures. In this section I examine in considerable detail the way various aims of selection developed and how they shaped the phenotype of animals across species and breeds, time, and country, but with a particular emphasis on North America. I do not deal with pet or hobbyist breeding as being distinct and separate from breeding for agricultural production. Instead I move freely across the breeding of pets, hobbyist animals, and farm stock. All pet and hobbyist breeding results from following the same theoretical and methodological procedures, and the same set of complicated selection aims. The differences rest on how impervious a breeder might be to incurring costs, and to characteristics which breeding is directed at. Breeding is breeding, regardless of what features are being bred for. The first chapter of the section deals with how specialization of purpose or use affected selection strategies, and as a consequence the way animal types changed. It will be apparent that shifting aspects of human society were intimately entangled with these developments.

Specialization: Greyhounds and Speed

One would initially think that specialization for speed would be a relatively simple concept, since speed is just speed, and therefore the aim of breeding for speed would be consistent through the ages. But speed can mean various things within the context of different societal needs and various cultural and technological conditions. Characteristics of breeding for speed can also be shown to reflect what adjustments selective methodology underwent with the shift from environmental to improvement breeding. A look at Greyhound dog breeding in England indicates that what people wanted from speed changed over time and in relation to how strongly the incentive to improvement breeding had taken hold. While I address the history of the English Greyhound, it is worth noting that the greyhound type of dog could be found in many European geographic areas for centuries, differing in features such as size and heaviness of fur coat, in accordance with its environment. It is also worth pointing out that an English and Scottish greyhound version clearly existed by 1200 in Britain.[1]

Breeders of the English Greyhound (by law only members of the nobility) from the thirteenth century until the eighteenth followed standard strategies of environmental breeding: maintaining the speed of the dogs by working with or against, as the case may be, environmental factors believed to direct inheritance. Ideas about generation, conception, and the balancing effects of certain strengths in males and females on the progeny with regard to the surroundings were important to systems of environmental breeding. Careful attention was given to the state of the heavens too; for example, the time breeding should take place. A bitch would not be mated during her heat until after the passage of the full moon. The result would be more males in the litter and better temperament. Over the centuries the aristocrats selected for various types of speed. Dogs bred to hunt deer were expected to have different speed skills, for example, from those in dogs designed to chase deer.[2]

By the early nineteenth century, the breeding of Greyhounds had started to shift both in terms of who bred the dogs and how the animals were bred. In 1831 parliament "democratized" Greyhound breeding; it would no longer be the priority of the elite. The move of the middle class into breeding and concurrently the sport of coursing took hold rapidly. Democratization of the breeding of Greyhounds seemed to go hand in hand with the improvement breeding principles that had emerged in the eighteenth century. Interest in improvement led to breeding Greyhounds, for example, with more rigid selection methods based on perceived hereditary characteristics of breeding pairs. The idea that environmental issues influenced inheritance had firmly taken a back seat by the latter half of the nineteenth century. In the years when the transition from environment to improvement breeding was taking place, the 1850s and 1860s, however, John Walsh (under the name of Stonehenge) wrote extensively about the correct way to breed Greyhounds and in doing so elucidated something of how uneven the transition actually was.

In his "General Principles of Breeding," written in 1864, Walsh noted that very little was known about the laws of inheritance. Even so, he was prepared to provide guidelines as to how selection practices should be carried out. Walsh clearly revealed, however, that vestiges of the past clung to his breeding theory: Lamarckism, for example, and the idea of acquired characteristics. "Acquired qualities of mind as well as of body may be transmitted by either parent," he stated. Competing with this concept, however, was his conviction that unknown forces or hereditary laws, and not the environment, drove how traits were inherited. Comments such as "The purer or less mixed the breed, the more likely it is to be transmitted in the same form as the parent" and "Bad as well as good qualities may be transmitted" indicate that Walsh believed inheritance was an issue outside environmental effects. He noted as well that, since "breeding 'in and in' cannot be shown to be injurious in wild animals," there is no reason to find it so in domestic animals. Most importantly, Walsh concluded "It will thus be seen that, though few, there are some broad landmarks which may serve to guide the breeder, and that by studying them he may hope to avoid the grievous errors so often made by those who think breeding is in all cases a complete lottery."[3] Evidently Walsh believed that breeding results proceeded from the interaction of genetic laws, even if these were not understood. Experimentation and judgment made it possible to bring about desired results. The new emphasis on selection outside the environment resulted in rapid specialization of the Greyhound for greater speeds.

From the beginning, the sports of coursing and racing were behind the breeding of these dogs. The regulation of English Greyhound racing began during the era of environmental breeding and as early as the reign of Elizabeth I. By the sixteenth century, dogs belonging to royalty and the nobility competed in formal coursing races for the pleasure of the elite. Greyhound racing and a system to support it as a commercial venture (as entertainment to be watched by the general public) did not arise until the late eighteenth century. The first Greyhound coursing club opened to the public in 1776, and by the early nineteenth century dog racing had attracted considerable attention. Specialization for speed under new breeding theory came increasingly to be directed by variation of locale and by differing coursing venues. The most important, and the one that would most engage the public, revolved around the Waterloo Cup, first held on Lord Molyneux's (Earl of Sefton) Altcar estate in 1836; the cup was won that year by the owner of the Waterloo Tavern in Liverpool. The type of Greyhound bred for coursing at the Altcar estate, where the Waterloo Cup has taken place ever since, became the best known.

Standardization of breeding for the terrain where the cup was held masked the fact that different Greyhound sports continued to exist outside that locale, and more successfully fitted a niche in those areas than the better-known version. Regulation of coursing over the years did not change that reality, although it orchestrated how versions of the sport would operate. The establishment of the National Coursing Club of England in 1858 began a more comprehensive way of organizing the sport of coursing dogs. Registration of Greyhounds in a public stud book evolved with the racing industry and was part of the increased structuring of the breeding industry under the purebred system, and the greater emphasis that selective mating under purebred breeding entailed. Interest in coursing, and the linkage of the nobility to Greyhounds, meant that some ancestry records had been kept privately as far back as the eighteenth century, but no public registry for Greyhounds in Britain existed until 1882, when the National Coursing Club required registration of dogs on the basis of parental recording in the Greyhound Stud Book for animals entering races.[4] New applicants that came from an unregistered parental background would be denied entry. Standardization of breeding through these various structural organizations did not, however, lead to a uniform type of speed in the dogs. Uniformity was not the dominant feature of Greyhounds after 1880. Speed, in effect, became a splintered specialization in accordance with the racing and coursing milieu that the dogs were bred for.

By 1900 three distinct greyhound skills developed for coursing – the Waterloo Cup variety (public match coursing), the private match coursing, and private hare hunting. The animals looked alike but had various racing abilities.[5] Greyhounds bred for public coursing differed from those for private coursing, and both differed from hare-hunting Greyhounds. Because the key variations were more behavioural than physical, they remained invisible for many people in England during the nineteenth century and later. Specialization might have appeared to lead to greater uniformity in the dogs' speed, but in fact it led to hidden differences. The real move towards greater speed homogeneity came with track racing, made possible by the use of a mechanical lure in the twentieth century.

The first artificial lure for Greyhound racing appeared in 1876, but mechanical lures were not in general use until after 1912, when an American, Owen Patrick Smith, invented a more workable one that could be used on a track. The popularity of track racing grew rapidly after that time in both Britain and the United States. By the late twentieth century, however, a movement against the sport had gathered strength. Various centres began to shut down tracks where racing took place. A centre of Greyhound racing on tracks in North America, for example, was Florida, which outlawed the sport as of 2020. Many tracks in the state closed earlier, that is in the spring of 2019 at the end of the year's racing season.

The breeding of Greyhounds shows how characteristics of breeding methodology changed over centuries yet remained focused on one type of specialization: speed. Specialization for speed, however, splintered into subsections of specialization as more effective approaches for dealing with heredity developed. The idea of specialization itself did not shift, but as methods to promote varying purposes did, the ramifications were more dramatic. Pedigree registration and the standardization of Greyhounds remained largely focused on the racing industry. When the purebred dog industry arose late in the nineteenth century under the Kennel Club structure, Greyhounds qualified for entry into that dog registry. The vast majority of Greyhounds, however, did not become part of the conformation show based system.

Specialization: Fancy Pigeon Breeding and Standardization of Beauty

One of the earliest animal types to be developed through specialization for improvement was the fancy pigeon. The trend towards improvement breeding of pigeons began during environmental breeding times, and from the beginning focused on beauty. (Pigeon breeding for speed followed a somewhat different path.) An ever greater drive for improvement with a focus on beauty would go on throughout the nineteenth century. Fancy pigeon breeding's particular significance to this story rests, however, not so much on the fact that breeding aims continued to be directed at beauty, but rather on the innovative way that beauty would be assessed. Few organizational structures for the breeding of animals would have more influence on how selection aims unfolded than that which evolved in the fancy pigeon world. Pigeon breeders created a written description of what was desired, organized on the basis of perceived beauty points, and thereby established the various aspects of beauty a breeder should be attempting to achieve. The result was a highly structured way of defining and verifying relative levels of beauty. The birds, in other words, could be evaluated against each other, and in a much more impersonal way than would result from various individual overall visual impressions. Breeding methodology itself played no role in how standards were designed.

This highly organized way of assessing beauty by assigning points for it in a relative fashion brought breeders of other species to study how pigeon breeding had become standardized. The orchestration of breeding around a written standard which judged phenotypic style would go on to affect other nineteenth-century breeding systems. The chicken industry's organization would be configured completely around beauty as set out by standards; in England by the Standard of Excellence and in the United States by the Standard of Perfection. The enormous popularity of chicken types developed within a recognized point system, and the fact that it aided judges in assessing excellence in the show ring, encouraged the purebred dog industry to embrace the pigeon strategy. Walsh had suggested written canine standards per breed as early as 1864 after F.C. Esquilant, a pigeon breeder, had explained how the numbered point system worked.[6] The English and American Kennel Clubs would adopt the idea when it came to recognizing established breeds of dogs.

Specialization: Chickens for Utility or Beauty

The introduction to the British and North American chicken world of the pigeon breeder attitude to standardization of beauty would have an enormous impact on how chicken breeders addressed improved utility specialization in the birds, meaning their ability to serve an egg and meat market. The conviction that improvement for beauty meant improvement in utility, namely that specialization for one led to specialization for the other, would become a major argument of chicken breeders. They pontificated on the utility use of their beauty-bred birds when trying to sell the animals to producing farmers. Beauty, however, in reality remained their primary concern. Classically described as "standardbreds" (sometimes as "thoroughbreds"), the birds conformed to written breed standards based on perceptions of beauty and were bred with that standard in mind. Quality was assessed only by how well the birds matched the beauty standards set for them. But as demand for utility in chickens grew over the nineteenth century, it increasingly behooved breeders to mask the fact that beauty and beauty alone drove their breeding decisions. They therefore argued ever more forcefully that beauty equalled utility. The prevailing and ongoing dominance of standardbred breeding in the chicken world, as established under the rulings of the Standards of Excellence (Britain) or Perfection (North

America), reinforced and encouraged this attitude that a fusion existed between beauty and utility aims.

The dichotomy presented by linking beauty with utility aroused considerable controversy as far as agricultural experts interested in improved utility on both sides of the Atlantic were concerned. Was beauty an issue to focus on at all, and why? Did breeding for fancy mean the same thing as breeding for utility? Either could be seen as an issue of improvement, but was it possible to accomplish both at the same time? When lip service was given to breeding for improvement of any utility use, but the standard actually focused only on beauty or fancy points, not any form of utility, could it correctly be argued that such animals were both useful and beautiful at the same time?[7]

The rise of the show ring as a means of judging improvement for beauty in the birds lay at the heart of the matter when it came to the beauty or utility issue. The organization of breeding for beauty was meant from the beginning to work in concert with and therefore support exhibition structures. The situation created an inbuilt and ongoing beauty versus utility dichotomy with respect to what purpose chickens served in both Britain and North America. By the 1870s it had become evident that concern with beauty for show purposes alone so dominated important early British poultry selective methods that many no longer even gave lip service to agricultural usefulness.[8] Farm experts in Britain blamed the rising obsession with beauty for an ongoing ruination of older, good producing lines.[9] They condemned the exhibition system, arguing that it had been a terrible mistake and should be abandoned.[10] Beauty breeding subsequently became completely detached from utility breeding in Britain, and by the 1890s utility breeders in that country had established their own organization to promote better production. They also imported American breeds to work with. Somewhat ironically, British breeders favoured using the working breeds that had been created in North America under an exhibition system that had originated in Britain.[11]

The beauty versus utility dichotomy (resulting from breeding for beauty as a way to achieve utility) arose within the North American chicken world as early as breeding for exhibition took hold. And by the 1860s agricultural experts and governments firmly believed that a show system for chickens would result in improved utility birds.[12] More poultry shows would probably help in the spread of improved stock, agreed the *Canadian Poultry Chronicle*.[13] Buy poultry from fancy breeders, the *Chronicle* advised. It doesn't cost more to keep good poultry than bad.[14] Exhibition breeders in Ontario argued that beautiful birds meant improved utility birds.[15] American breeders concurred. An important breeder, U.R. Fishel of Indiana, explained the situation by describing how the White Plymouth Rock fitted into the show and farm worlds. (The white variety arose from the hatching eggs of the Barred Plymouth Rock variety in 1875, when O.F. Frost of Monmouth, Maine found he had white chicks from his barred eggs.[16] White Rocks had all the good qualities of the Barred Rocks.)[17] "Not only has [the White Rock] been bred for fancy points, but the utility part of the breed has been retained and carefully looked after until today the breed ranks first as egg producers, while as a market fowl there is no breed to compare with them," he stated. Fishel emphasized his success in producing top quality White Rocks with both fancy and utility features. "I remember when the U.R. Fishel White Plymouth Rocks were first introduced," he reminisced just after 1900; "people realized that I was striving hard to give them a fancy fowl that was also a business fowl. My combining both beauty and utility in my strain of White Plymouth Rocks has convinced the poultrymen the world over that it pays to breed a variety of fowls that can fill any place where a chicken is wanted."[18] As late as the 1920s, Fishel repeated that his concern was for beauty and utility, and added that he had succeeded in making his stock both more beautiful and more useful.[19]

By the late 1880s, in spite of ongoing claims of breeders like Fishel that beauty and use were combined in exhibition breeding, the idea that shows successfully encouraged the rise of better farm chickens no longer attracted the same general public acceptance that it had in the late 1860s. People increasingly questioned views held by breeders like Fishel, and wondered as well about the effects of the show system on agricultural interests. The Mark Lane *Express*, an English-based journal, spoke out strongly about the failure of the show system to promote useful farm birds in 1888. "The fancier who minces the matter, preferring to allow the world to continue to believe that exhibitions instruct and improve the people in a particular direction is insincere. In answer to the question, What has the poultry fancy done for profitable poultry? we must answer, clearly enough, nothing."[20] The *Canadian Poultry Review* agreed with the position taken by the *Express*. Poultry exhibitions were designed to help farmers, not fanciers, an article pointed out in 1892, but since farmers rarely went to shows focused on beauty points, they in fact learned nothing.[21] The apparent focus on beauty made the funding of poultry shows by government increasingly contentious in both Canada and the United States. "Feathers count and *feathers only*," the *Farmer's Advocate* fumed in 1900, proclaiming they were the chief object of shows. Look at such breeds as the "football-haired Polish," the journal pointed out. Fanciers produced breeds that were "a curse to any farmer or practical poultryman," it concluded.[22]

John Dryden, the Ontario minister of agriculture, explained to breeders that the state support of shows was meant to encourage a better understanding among farmers of what constituted superior and improved poultry. Addressing the Poultry Association of Ontario in 1894, he told members that the government did not fund shows in order simply to provide breeders with prizes. Farmers did not see the colour of a feather as evidence of superior breeding. Utility was what they wanted. Dryden also believed that fanciers did little to help farmers understand how to breed or care for poultry in a more satisfactory way.[23] The thorny problem of state involvement with prize money for exhibition fowl that clearly did not supply farms with useful birds bothered Americans too.[24] Government funding of breeder activity which worked off a show system makes it clear, however, that the state looked to the breeders as experts and therefore sought their guidance on how best to support and encourage superior agricultural breeding practices. The exhibition system triggered similar debates about the impact of shows on the breeding of purebred horses and cattle.[25] The direct relationship of showing to breeding remained most strident, however, within the standardbred poultry world, because the show system and emphasis on breeding for beauty in it were two sides of the same coin. Suggesting that the show system for beauty resulted in birds equally useful for utility could not hide the reality that beauty was the true base of the system.

One wonders if the situation would have been different if purebred breeding had undermined the beauty breeding which so dominated the chicken world. Purebred breeding at least offered ways of advancing characteristics not related to phenotypic beauty, selection on the basis of perceived productivity being one. The method allowed for flexibility along these lines because the purebred system rested primarily on the recording of pedigrees and not on written beauty standards. Ancestry, not beauty, was the dictator of how selection under purebred breeding had to proceed. (Purebred breeding and standardbred breeding might function together, as is the case in the Kennel Club system. Such a union, however, has done little to defuse the emphasis on beauty as the primary driver in show dog breeding.)

There had, in fact, been some pressure to make poultry breeding fit with prevailing purebred standards. In 1870 the *Canadian Poultry Chronicle* openly campaigned for a public registry system for chickens in order to make them truly qualify as purebred. "Poultry with a registered pedigree would be a novelty, yet we see no reason why the novelty should not exist; other livestock have their Pedigree-Book, and why not poultry too?" the paper asked. Pedigrees would solve another problem too, the journal argued, namely what the origin of evolving breeds actually was. "Is the origin [of many American breeds] to remain buried in obscurity [as is true in Britain] as it now apparently is? Surely not," remarked the *Chronicle*.[26] In 1874 the *Poultry World* in the United States tried to get support for a registry which would pedigree poultry, but ridicule from other poultry journals killed the idea.[27] Public recording would not spread to countries beyond Canada, even though there was considerable admiration for the plan in the poultry world. Breeders and government officials in both Britain and the United States, for example, at least noted the Canadian developments with interest. The editor of a British journal, C.A. House, greatly admired this initiative.[28] Americans were even more impressed.[29] "The registration of chickens in an official record book, so as to afford a legitimate basis for tracing pedigrees, is something new in the poultry world, although it has long been established" for other livestock, stated the *American Poultry Journal*.

> Now comes the Canadian government with the announcement that it has granted to poultry breeders the right to register purebred chickens in national registration records. This is a step toward "blue blood" and a "poultry aristocracy." The National Poultry Record Association has been organized in Canada and has opened a registration book to all Canadian breeders of [thoroughbred] fowls. Mongrels cannot be registered.[30]

The registry structure of purebred breeding did not take hold in any broad way throughout the poultry world. The ethos of standardbred breeding remained in force, making allegiance to a system that promoted only beauty more entrenched. The potential that public recording at least might have offered for advancing different selection aims would, therefore, never be in place. In the end that situation, in concert with others, encouraged the development of other avenues for improved utility chicken breeding. While many factors went into why the takeover of chicken breeding for table eggs by the corn companies happened, the profound concern with beauty that the American Poultry Association promoted played a role in that revolution.

Specialization and the Impact of Technology: Dairy Cattle Breeding in Canada and the Netherlands

Specialization for utility in animals is more normally seen, not as an issue of beauty's fusion with utility as was the case in nineteenth- and early twentieth-century North American chickens, but rather as a concern with making animals perform well in service of different industry purposes. As livestock industries became more commercially viable, especially under the impact of innovative technology, a significant question would emerge: could the same animals serve two industries equally well, or should they be specialized for one only? In other words, should they be bred for dual-purpose use or single-purpose use? With respect to chickens, the purpose breeding trouble erupted over the 1930s and 1940s when a division between meat-producing (broiler) birds and table-egg-laying birds began to evolve. Purpose matters occurred earlier in cattle breeding, coming under especially important pressure from changing technology after 1870. The rise of cheese and butter factories, which increased the demand for dairy products, initiated a beef or dairy specialization dilemma in a way that had not been so apparent earlier. The quandary in various countries became how or whether to emphasize beef or dairy specialization in order to meet the new conditions.

The response of Canadian and Dutch dairy cattle breeders to the situation over the late nineteenth and early twentieth centuries provides specific examples of how the purpose predicament was addressed because of pressure from changing technologies. Historically, attitudes to cattle uses had developed differently in Canada and the Netherlands, thereby laying divergent foundations for what type of cattle would initially work with the new technologies. Canadians had tended to concentrate their breeding efforts on improving beef production more efficiently, while the Dutch had tended to select for improved dairy production. With the advent of cheese factories, Dutch interest in dairy qualities meant their cows would fit the new technology reasonably well, and certainly better than stock in Canada where beef breeding reigned. The rise of factories for the making of first cheese and then butter clearly created a difficult state of affairs in Canada because selection for beef, reflecting eighteenth- and nineteenth-century developments in Britain, had long been favoured by Canadian breeders. Societal transitions in Britain had shaped cattle breeding in Canada.

Both British urbanization and industrialization had encouraged an increased demand for meat in that country, and the British purebred breeding system would be based on specializing "beefing" characteristics of cattle. (The trend in Britain to breeding for beef had originated with Bakewell, as we have seen, and would be further promoted by Bates and his Shorthorns.) When purebred breeding entered Canada, then, it naturally related closely to beef breeding, and in fact the emphasis took greater hold in North America than it had in Britain.[31] The purebred industry in Canada came to be dominated by beef cattle and their breeders. (Shorthorns, a beef breed, greatly outnumbered all other breeds.) Few purebred dairy cattle existed in the country.[32] The concurrent British and North American belief that cattle were naturally better milkers than beefers led agricultural experts and farmers alike in Canada to link the concept of purebred improvement closely to beefing characteristics.[33] As the *Farmer's Advocate* stated in 1887, Canada's native cows were unsurpassed milk producers but were poor beef producers.[34]

I review Canada's approach to the matter of purpose breeding of cattle to serve cheese and butter factories in this predominantly beef world by assessing Ontario's experience with the problem. The province's rich documentation, particularly the five-volume report of the Ontario Agricultural Commission (released in 1881), commentary in the farm press, and various government documents provide direct testimony with regard to how cattle breeding should proceed. It becomes clear from these sources that the two major groups of people interested in breeding for the dairy, namely purebred breeders (but often agricultural experts as well) and ordinary farmers practising dairying, held divergent views on how to handle the predicament.[35] The first faction argued for dual-purpose production through the use of beef-oriented cattle for beef and dairying. Purebred cattle in Ontario might be overwhelmingly specialized for beef, but their owners and agricultural experts insisted that the animals fitted beautifully with systems of dual-purpose farming. Agricultural experts and purebred breeders supported that position on the basis that all cows (therefore beef cows too) were by nature good milkers.[36] Farmers took a different view. They had come quite quickly to believe that true dual-purpose farming with cattle was not the way to go because different animals were needed to perform successfully in the beef and dairy industries.[37] Furthermore, while they saw beef cattle as fitting well with beef farming, they did not see them as useful in the dairy.

On top of that situation, they did not link any specialized breeding with dairying. Ordinary cows with no specialized breeding were considered the best animals for the dairy industry. As early as 1869, the Agriculture and Arts Association (the government body supporting agriculture at the time in Ontario) was told that "[t]here [seemed] to be an idea prevalent with many of our dairymen that any kind of stock or cows [would] answer the purposes of a dairy."[38] When Ontario farmers undertook beef production, as they did in considerable numbers throughout the 1870s and into the early 1880s, they actively selected for beefing characteristics and were even prepared to incur at least some purebred genetic "improvement" of their herds in order to increase that beefiness. The underlying conflict over how specialization should function in cattle operations remained hidden as long as farmers practised beef farming to any great extent. But when they abandoned beef farming in ever greater numbers and turned to dairying, it became obvious that they rejected the idea of dual-purpose cattle and the need for specialization in dairy cows. In the process, farmers tended to give up any breeding activity relating to cattle as well.

Characteristics which would increasingly dominate dairying after the rise of factory cheese could be seen as early as 1880. As a witness on dairy affairs in Ontario, Thomas Ballantyne, stated that year to members of the agricultural commission, "Dairymen, as a rule, do not consider it profitable to raise their own stock." He added that he himself would advise farmers not to breed or rear their own dairy cows. "If I were dairying I would not think of raising my stock. I would sell the cows when they became useless, and always be on the lookout for good milkers, as a good cow will pay for herself in one season," he said.[39] Another dairyman, D.M. Macpherson, confirmed the practice of buying replacement cows rather than raising them. "I do not raise many calves, but supply myself by purchasing," he stated to the commissioners.[40] In effect, dairy farmers abandoned specialized beef breeding, purebred breeding, and to some degree even breeding itself with the increased mechanization of cheese production. When Ontario farmers turned in greater numbers to dairying they also emphasized other practices. Farmers often killed dairy calves at birth.

By not raising most calves from their dairy cows for beef purposes, farmers confirmed an avoidance of any form of dual-purpose production. The action also denoted an evading of breeding for the dairy. The calf-killing practice began in conjunction with factory cheese manufacturing as early as 1870. A dairyman, C.A. Matheson, explained the circumstances to the members of the Ontario Agricultural Commission. His district had always been a dairy district where primarily butter had been made on the farm. The arrival of cheese factories entirely changed the picture. Butter making was dropped, milk from the cows was sent to the cheese factories, and calves were killed at birth. Matheson said, "the farmers [used to raise] all their own calves; but in the last eight or ten years a large number of cheese factories have been opened. [Farmers now no longer make butter, ship milk to the cheese factories instead, and] generally kill their calves. The consequence is that the stock is deteriorating [and the number of animals is declining] ... The people who are dairying [for these cheese factories] ... attempt to get all the milk they can, and kill off nearly all the calves ... The cattle from which the cheese factories are supplied are generally good common native milkers," he added, but implied that increasingly there was a shortage of them.[41]

It was clear by 1883 that the calf-killing practice had become quite extensive in the province. At least two hundred thousand calves were killed at birth in Ontario that year, and markets were flooded with slaughter calves less than four weeks old.[42] An alarmed Shorthorn breeder argued that single dairy purpose "leads to that cruel and revolting practice of slaughtering all, or nearly all, the calves at birth. Much is said these days about making home attractive to the boys on the farm. Is it any wonder that a boy of spirit and refinement should want to get away from those yearly scenes of carnage and bloodshed! It clashes with all our preconceived ideas of the laws of the creator."[43] In an article called "Protest against Calf Slaughter," the *Farmer's Advocate* mourned that "[i]n large districts of the country, this calf murder goes on every spring. Some will blame the low price of beef, others the cheese factory system, for this slaughter; but is it not wasteful and slovenly?"[44] The trend to calf killing continued and gathered strength wherever a greater emphasis on dairying took place.

In spite of extensive calf killing and the expansion of dairying under the impetus of technology, some farmers could appear to be following the advice of the purebred breeders. If, however, farmers ran cattle operations that seemed to reflect dual-purpose production, in reality they concentrated on one specialization only. They ran the other for small by-product or supplementary reasons. They also used different animals to serve each purpose. When a farmer pursued dairying, his primary herd would comprise milkers, but he might also keep separately a few beef cows in order to raise their calves for beef. If a farmer focused on beef farming, he could supplement this income by having a few ordinary cows for dairying in order to produce milk. In other words, farmers straddled the line between the two specializations by making one subservient to the other and using different cows, generally speaking, for production. One way to see this pattern is to note remarks made in reports in the early 1880s to the Ontario government. The government allocated prizes to farms from 1882 to 1893 thought to be examples of excellence, and in doing so revealed how individual farmers operated in the province. Reference was frequently made about two types of cattle on a farm in the transition period. Note the detailed emphasis on specialized purebred breeding for beef, and the separate use of general non-purebred cows for the dairy in a 1882 report on one farm.

> There are at this time 82 head of cattle [on this farm]; 37 of these are pedigreed Shorthorns, and 20 cows kept for dairy purposes, the balance

> being young stock of different ages, amongst which are a good number of fine fleshy steers for fattening this winter – just the sort of stock for making good shippers next spring. The thoroughbreds are a fine lot, good pedigrees and good animals ... Taken together, it is a very fine herd of Shorthorns, both as regards breeding and also in respect of the individual merits of the animals ... The dairy stock, as already said, comprises 20 cows. These cows are of the ordinary run of stock ...[45]

A major question left unanswered here is what happened to the calves of the twenty milch cows. The young stock of the beef thoroughbreds would be fed out for beef. This was a beef specialization farm, possibly using dairy calves to some unknown degree as a by-product of dairying to augment the beef operation. More likely, however, calf killing was practised extensively. It is worth noting that over the years in reports for these prize farms it appeared to be assumed that farmers killed dairy calves at birth, because in locations where the practice was not followed, inspectors went out of their way to report it. No such comment was made with respect to this farm.

While the feeding of dairy calves for beef (often described as "factory calves" which were "cheesed" out of their milk)[46] might have been done to a limited degree in the 1880s, the effect of these surviving dairy calves on the beef market became dramatic after 1890 when specialized beef operations went into serious decline. There were a number of reasons for the reduction of beef farming and the tendency of farmers to start into dairying. To begin with, the beef cattle industry was subject to unpleasant volatility in income. That volatility was embedded in production methods and in marketing systems over which farmers had little control. In contrast, dairying offered a more stable income. The financial support of governments for dairying (via cold storage, funded transportation for dairy products, and the extension of dairying education) made that industry even more attractive. Dairying became so pervasive in Ontario after 1900 that much of beef production had in fact become a by-product of the dairy industry.[47] The calves generated by dairy farmers began in greater numbers (proportionately speaking, compared to beef calves) to play a significant part in the feeder sector of the beef industry. As feeder farmers found it harder and harder to find beef calves from the declining number of cow/calf operators, dairy calves became a greater factor in the beef industry's feeder sector.

Persistent calf killing and the ongoing reluctance of dairymen to generate their stock through breeding might have kept the actual number of dairy stock available limited, but a shortage of beef oriented calves at the same time aggravated the situation.[48] It was clearly evident as early as 1897 that the number of animals serving the beef industry in Ontario had dropped and that the quality of steers on the market had become inferior.[49] Dairy oriented calves, even if in limited supply, had come by percentage to dominate the feeder structure. Feeder farmers quickly found it unprofitable to fatten such stock and began to stop running any beef operations. The general shortage of feeder stock and a decline in feeder outfits ultimately resulted in a decrease of meat available for the consumer. The existence of an underlying emphasis on one specialization (dairying) over the other (beef) continued to underlie the feeder cattle problem and therefore the beef industry situation. It escaped no one that beef industry conditions reflected the fact that cattle farming in Ontario had become primarily focused on dairying, in spite of the fact that one farm might generate products relating to both beef and dairy.

Unimproved dairy cows, it would soon be proven, were no better for the dairy industry than dairy purpose stock was for the beef industry. Better feeding did result in the rise of milk production over the 1890s from its level of three thousand pounds per cow a year, but nowhere near the five thousand pound mark, estimated in 1895 as being what was needed per year for profitability. The actual quality of dairy cattle did not improve either. "The breeding of [dairy] class cattle is not considered so very important. A high standard of breeding is, in most cases, overlooked by the [dairy] farmer," the *Advocate* pointed out as late as 1909.[50] The subsequent recognition by farmers that milk yields from such cows could not adequately sustain dairy farming, however, would ultimately bring about a reorientation of attitudes towards specialized and therefore perceived improved breeding, especially after 1915.[51] The turning of the tide in favour of specialized purebred dairy cattle for better production came with studies done by the Ontario Agricultural College, which confirmed the importance of specialized cattle (through purebred breeding) for profitability in dairying. Farm size and even feed costs, the studies showed, were not as significant as the level of dairy specialization quality in the livestock for profitability.[52] (Purebred cows in Ontario were capable of sixteen thousand pounds a year at that time.)

The acute labour shortage on farms during the First World War helped to trigger a willingness to change. Farmers needed superior production with fewer animals. They began in increasing numbers after 1918 to use Holstein cattle. Specialized breeding was now linked by Ontario farmers to dairy qualities as well as beef qualities. By 1920 Holstein breeders reported more ownership transfers than the Shorthorn breeders did, and membership in the Holstein Association was nearly as high as that of the Shorthorn Association.[53] Dairy farmers in Ontario remained true to their fundamental desire to farm with cattle in a single purpose focused way when they commenced in greater numbers to use purebred, specialized dairy genetics. Beef as a by-product of the intensified dairy industry, however, continued to be a problem and to some degree is still with us today. While beef oriented animals play the most significant role in the modern beef industry, dairy beef is at least part of the story. The raising of dairy calves and the nature of the veal market have also become ethical issues, even if calf killing went into decline.[54]

The Ontario situation with respect to dairy cattle contrasted sharply with that in the Netherlands over the years between 1880 and 1920. The well-known Friesian Black and White had been bred single-purpose dairy for centuries by the 1880s and therefore seamlessly worked with the new technology. During the 1890s there was an intensification of specializing for dairy qualities in the Friesians in response to the rise of cheese factories and creameries. Breeders strove for even greater intensification of dairy qualities, particularly in certain provinces such as Friesland and North Holland. Cattle took on even stronger dairy characteristics as their milk yield increased. By the late nineteenth century, Dutch cattle had come to look like the more modern Holstein, a North American derivative of the Friesian. Cows were tall, leggy, narrow chested, deep bodied, and gaunt. They were known in Britain, where beefier animals dominated, as "milking machines." Change was in the wind, however, for cattle breeding in the Netherlands early in the twentieth century. The threat of bovine tuberculosis, which gathered momentum at the end of the nineteenth century, brought about a reorientation to dairy cattle breeding in that country.[55] At the same time that Canadian dairymen showed signs of becoming interested in specialized breeding for dairying, Dutch farmers started to reduce their focus on breeding of single-purpose dairying. They began a process of introducing beef or robust characteristics to the cattle at the same time that Canadians initiated the move to lessen beefing qualities in dairy cattle.

Bovine TB, recognized as a serious international threat by the late 1890s, provoked various theories about its nature and how to control it. Confusion over contagion, infection via miasma, and sanitation was evident in the contemporary conviction that tuberculosis was a particular menace to purebred cattle. Studies in some parts of the world did indicate that the relationship of the disease to purebred stock could be as high as 100 per cent.[56] The prevalence of the disease in purebred herds, which tended to be more closely housed and to share bedding and drinking troughs, made it unclear to breeders whether sanitation or contagion was the source of the disease. (It would soon be known that the disease was passed from one animal to another mostly by aerosol exchange of droplets, clearly more likely when cattle were kept in close proximity to one another.) The system of soiling (stall, rather than pasture, feeding of green fodder in summer) also encouraged the spread of TB, although the connection between soiling and the presence of TB did not seem to be evident at the time. John G. Rutherford, who became veterinary general for Canada in 1902 and later also livestock commissioner, claimed that Bow Park (the large Shorthorn breeding operation mentioned at the beginning of the introduction to this book) was the "distributing centre for the whole of western Ontario of bovine tuberculosis" and for many parts of the Midwestern United States as well.[57] Because soiling was practised at Bow Park, the herd almost certainly contained a high proportion of tuberculosis at least partially as a result, because contagion spread more readily under these conditions than under pasturing. It was clear as well from numerous studies in the United States over the late nineteenth century that bovine TB was also commonly seen in dairy herds; again animals more closely housed and not kept on open pastures.[58]

The idea that overly specialized dairy cows, owing to the excessively thin and bony characteristics of the phenotype (physical looks), were susceptible to bovine TB led Dutch dairymen and agricultural experts in the Netherlands to associate the extreme dairy type of the contemporary Friesian with a propensity to develop TB. The reaction of breeders was to select for more robust, beefier animals, also believed to be more pleasant to the eye in terms of beauty. The new dual-purpose type stock attracted buyers, particularly in Germany and Britain, where beefier animals were preferred for the dairy. In reality the Dutch breeders were not trying to create a dual-purpose breed. They simply believed that the newer form, although it sacrificed milk yield levels, was healthier and more serviceable generally. Dutch cattle enjoyed a heyday as a result of these changes up to the 1950s. (The older 1890s type had provided the backbone for North American breeding of Holsteins. The modern beefier Friesian's market was not North America.) This situation contrasted sharply with that in North America, where TB had little to no effect on how dairy stock was bred, even if efforts to control the spread of TB commanded a great deal of attention. The move in Canada to breeding more, not less, specialized dairy cattle ultimately did dovetail with the increased attention to TB in North America. But since Canadian dairy herds generally lacked the degree of specialization found in Dutch cattle for a considerable length of time, and since beef purebred herds were just as likely to have TB, Canadians did not tend to see specialization as an issue of TB. Other problems, such as war shortages, led breeders to increasingly emphasize dairy characteristics in the evolving Holstein at a time when Dutch cattle had moved the other way.

In Ontario, while selection for beef took precedence over selection for dairy characteristics, agricultural experts and farmers were not divided in opinion over the need to breed for beef. The divide rested on the issue of purpose or use in cattle: dairying in a dual-purpose way using beef cows versus dairying in a single-purpose way using unspecialized cows. Breeding for dairy qualities did not take hold in this traditional beef breeding country for a considerable length of time. Instead, efforts at improving the output of dairy products rested on calf killing, the continued use of cows inferior in milking qualities, and the avoidance of breeding itself. No such divided purpose hampered the breeding of cows for dairy qualities in the Netherlands, where cattle had always been specialized for the dairy (with beef production playing only a secondary and terminal role). In the end, however, a curious reversal with respect to beef specialization took place in Canadian and Dutch views on dairy cattle breeding. Dairy qualities became ever more important in Canadian cattle while beef related qualities became more desirable in Dutch dairy cattle.

Industrialization and the Specialization of Horses for Traction Needs

Selection patterns applied to horses on North American farms in the late nineteenth and early twentieth century illustrate another specialization issue. In this case it was a matter of size, shape, and weight in the working horse. The demand for different animals specialized by weight and size emerged from various traction needs emanating out of industrial and urban growth, not agriculture, and would drive how specialization in horse breeding evolved by the late nineteenth century.[59] There seemed over the years to be an increasing shortage of useful horses to serve these divergent traction markets in both North America and Europe. Royal commissions were called a number of times in Britain over the late nineteenth century in efforts at understanding why the situation existed in that country. A primary reason, it appeared, was that it took longer to change the phenotype of the horse than for shifting industrial needs to evolve. Enough horses of different sizes and weights simply did not exist at any one time. A review of how horses were bred in North America over the late nineteenth and early twentieth centuries, when the principal breeders of working horses were farmers who produced the animals for their use and for work off farms, reveals that other factors also explained that shortage. The farmer's horse, called a "chunk," or a general-purpose animal, in both Canada and the United States, served all markets for traction use.

For agricultural work, farmers in North America favoured a horse that belonged to neither the excessively specialized light nor the heavy draft type, an animal also not associated with the idea of breed. A move to greater specialization for industrial needs, combined with the rise of purebred heavy Clydesdales and Percherons (a subject which will be discussed in more detail in chapter 8), complicated the situation. How well, the question became, could the agricultural horse serve the new industrial and urban traction needs, especially in light of the presence of the heavier drafts? Endless conflicting views emerged over these questions. It became increasingly important, too, to define what an agricultural horse actually was.

Various definitions found in the farm press over the last part of the nineteenth and early part of the twentieth century attempted to describe what it meant to call a horse a "chunk" or a general-purpose horse. The Ontario Agricultural Commission described a general-purpose horse in 1880 as an animal that "is a light horse that can work on the farm and drive about 12 miles per hour on the road."[60] In the United States, the *Breeder's Gazette* in 1882 spoke of a medium-sized horse that made a "class of useful horses that may be called the farmer's horse."[61] In 1905 the *Farmer's Advocate* defined a general-purpose horse as "one that can be well utilized in ordinary farm work of all kinds and can also do a limited amount of road work." A horse defined as a good "chunk" was an animal "standing 15 to 16 hands high, weighing from 1,100 to 1,400 pounds, compactly built, with good feet and legs, tractable, lively disposition, a good clean, rapid way of going at walk or trot."[62] He was "nothing but a small drafter."[63]

Specialization ideas, however, soon demanded that horses sold off farms fit into certain types. The farmer's horse came increasingly to be known as the no-purpose horse, especially in Britain, where greater specialization to light and heavy horses existed earlier than in North America.[64] The hegemony of the Thoroughbred and the use of purebred heavy drafters by British farmers seemed to have made the crossbred, medium sized or even small work animal somewhat redundant. The fact that the general-purpose agricultural horse did not fit clearly into any off-farm market created a fundamental problem for the horse industry. Farmers tried to breed general-purpose animals for their needs primarily and to provide off-farm markets with stock from that pool of farm horses. But this approach made agricultural experts (and purebred heavy horse importers and breeders) unhappy with the quality of horses found in the marketplace.

Increasingly, horses wanted off the farm represented a variety of distinct classes which often the standard chunk could not fill. A document published in the United States by the Bureau of Animal Industry in 1901 explains horse classification for market purposes. A horse for urban use was listed as the "vanner," which worked at a walk, was a compact draft type of 1,600 to 1,800 pounds, and was wanted in the export market for city use. A vanner was clearly much bigger and heavier than a farm chunk. Other draft types more closely resembled a chunk, but were thought to be clearly distinct from the general-purpose farm horse. These city drafts worked at a trot and were described as the "expresser" (extremely desirable and weighing 1,250 to 1,500 pounds) and the "busser" (the omnibus horse, of 1,200 to 1,400 pounds, compact and rugged): "He [answered], to some extent, the call for a general purpose horse, but he should not be confused with the horse quoted as 'general-purpose' in market reports." Bussers were in short supply, given the demand for them, while "trammers" were smaller, plainer bussers and were used in European cities to pull trams. Market types listed in the American Agricultural Department publication of 1901 seemed to match those in Canada: the same article was released in the Canadian farm press, under the heading "The Kind of Horses the Market Demands."[65] Horses bred on farms were selected by weight to fit these different types of work.

The best way to produce animals for this complicated city market, as well as the general-purpose or agricultural horse, stimulated debate in the farm press. Over the years a mass of conflicting theories were put forward in the farm press in which farmers were told to breed heavy to light, light to light, and heavy to heavy. Farmers were, also confusingly, told that these conflicting practices produced both general-purpose and specialized horses. But at the same time the press often informed farmers that no such thing as a general-purpose horse existed. Views on how to breed chunk types in particular triggered completely ambiguous statements such as the following: The practice of using heavy stallions on light mares has resulted in many poor horses.[66] The heavy horse (namely animals with Clydesdale, Shire, or Percheron blood) should be crossed on the Thoroughbred types to produce strong working horses.[67]

Agricultural experts often argued that farmers should not be breeding for the chunk type at all, even if it was a good agricultural horse. It was not initially always clear, though, whether farmers were being told that they should be breeding for their own needs and selling leftover horses for city use, or that they should concentrate on city horses and use leftovers on the farm. How crossbreeding of purebreds or the development of new lines fitted into this story was rarely, if ever, addressed by the farm press. The problem was generally approached simply as one of weight. As demand for horses off the farm grew, the market focus of advice to farmers became clearer: experts increasingly exhorted farmers to produce for outside needs, arguing that any horse could serve on the farm. As early as 1878 this thought was put forward. The *Farmer's Advocate* stated: "Now farmers normally say they are breeding for themselves and their own use and want general-purpose horses. But they will sell those horses quickly if the need or opportunity arises. So why not simply breed for sale and not for use?"[68] The *Gazette* reminded farmers in 1882 that it was they who supplied the whole market for horses, and they should focus on more than just the production of agricultural horses.[69]

The American press published farmers' reactions to the unrelenting advice put forward on how and why they should breed horses, and also on the pressure to rely on purebreds, preferably those from the heavy draft breeds. Correspondence sent to the *Gazette* clearly showed that American farmers not only preferred to breed the light general-purpose horse but also resented pressure to use either heavy drafts or purebreds. One man wrote to the *Breeder's Gazette*, putting it this way: "After all has been said, and in spite of the ridicule and scoffing of the 'special-purpose' men, the horse best adapted to the needs of … farmers is what we call the general-purpose horse."[70] A man who understood the promotional thinking behind heavy purebred breeder messages had an answer for them: farmers needed the original chunk, the all-purpose horse that was not of huge draft size. "The all-purpose horse is the only horse we need and the horse that brings in the most money [too]," he wrote.[71] When one subscriber wrote in to state that the 1,100-pound horse served as a better all-purpose horse than the 1,600-pound animal, he was answered with the argument that it was a marketing issue.[72] The *Gazette* continued to reiterate that sentiment: all horses should reflect what the general horse market wanted. Horses should always be bred for the off-farm trade. In the late 1890s, before the advent of the horseless carriage, the best markets were either for good light harness animals or for very heavy quality drafts. Farmers should, therefore, not focus on breeding the intermediate-sized general-purpose horses, and therefore not breed specifically for horses to be used on the farm.[73]

One reader fumed over these arguments that farmers should focus more on specialization for various off-farm needs: "Eight or ten years ago we were advised to raise horses – draft horse, coacher and trotters. Many of us did so and have become practically bankrupt." Buyers kept demanding new things. "A few years ago a well-formed, blocky, 1,400 lb horse was a draft horse; now he is only a chunk and worth forty to fifty dollars. A [2 ½ minute trotting] horse was a trotter; now he is despised on the county fair race-track." No one near me, the writer added, bred horses any more unless he wanted a colt himself. He bred only for a general-purpose horse, the one he could sell to his neighbours.[74] For the *Gazette*, this type of thinking had been a major cause of the depressed horse market of the 1890s. Poor quality stock had glutted the market as a result of these "haphazard" breeding strategies.[75] In other words, the horse market continued to carry a large number of generalized, poorly specialized animals, in spite of the fact that demand called for ever greater distinctive types.

Electric tramways, bicycles, and horseless carriages had undermined the market for all lighter horses by 1900, in such a way that it was hard to see how it could recover. Farmers were not encouraged to breed them. At least that form of specialization was no longer in demand. The need for various versions of the heavy horse, however, continued unabated. After 1900 the press argued that all horse breeding on farms should be directed at the heavy horse, even if some of the animals were destined to work on the farm. Comments written between 1900 and 1914 in the Canadian farm press questioned the advisability of breeding any general-purpose horses in an increasingly heavy draft equine world. Since there is no longer a market for any horse of the general-purpose type, one writer opined, why encourage the breeding of such horses?[76] Farmers could and should breed for use on the farm and for sales purposes by using the pure drafts, Clyde or Shire.[77] Comments to the effect that the farm chunk was not desired in any off-farm trade, and that the heavy drafter was wanted, meant it only made sense that farmers breed and also use heavy horses.[78] The demand for heavy drafters made them the horse the farmer should breed.[79] "There are a lot of odd jobs and regular doings [at] which the light type of drafter excels the very heavy animal on the farm," it was often admitted. But the problem was that, when selling a horse, weight became extremely important. General-purpose horses commanded no money. "The demand is for heavy horses. They do the farm work almost, if not quite, as well, and at practically the same cost, as the lighter drafter horses." Therefore, farmers should breed heavy drafters. "The cry of the city is for the massive draft animal. It is this type of horse which tops the market … Therefore, all things considered, the heavy drafter, and preferably a purebred, is the horse for the farm."[80] Sometimes farmers did follow the advice of the journals and used specialized horse types designed to serve in the off-farm markets. In the United States, farmers were known to deliberately breed with outside markets in mind, and they farmed with whatever was left after sales.[81]

Increasingly technology, in the form of gasoline engines to be used on farms (primarily tractors), within cities, and finally in industry made the picture look murky when it came to the breeding of any horses. Would heavy horses soon be redundant? Would trucks take over the work of heavy horses, the way cars had taken over the horse and buggy? No one knew, the *Advocate* admitted in 1915.[82] By 1918 the situation looked different and, if anything, bleaker for horses. Even while bemoaning the lack of appreciation for the heavier horse's capacity to serve, *Farm and Dairy* was forced to state that the new technology, particularly the internal gasoline combustion engine, might mean the end for the workhorse at some point in the near future. Increasing mechanization of traction left the heavy draft horse as the main survivor, even if somewhat shakily by 1920, of the working horse world. Because there were still markets for the type off the farm, farmers became more inclined to breed the heavy drafter, or what might be described as a heavier chunk, for use on the farm as well. The farm horse of the 1950s would look more like the classic Clyde, or Percheron, even if it was a crossbred animal.[83] Chunk had merged into, or with, the heavy draft horse which served on farms until the mid-twentieth century. Technology off the farm had led to the ever heavier horse serving any horse market that was left.

How well horses were able to fit specialized work for specific purpose (farmers never did breed for the designated jobs of vanners, expressers, or bussers) is not known beyond the general complaints that the animals did not do so. Horses employed in cities and industry came from a pool of animals generated on farms; in most cases from animals bred for farm purposes but occasionally from equine operations where farmers contented themselves with using stock left over from industrial sales. The rapidity with which traction needs developed and splintered made it difficult, if not impossible, to keep up with the creation of specialized animals to match need, regardless of farmers' propensity to focus on breeding for farm use. The inability to react to change in fact probably encouraged them to continue simply breeding for farm use. The overall effect of traction demands on the phenotype of horses would, however, be dramatic. Industry might have failed to splinter haulage type to any large degree, but it drove trends in the general horse population towards heavier animals – for farm use or off-farm use. In the end traction technology would eliminate the use of horses for any work of that nature.

While the problem of selection for purpose or various uses was a major issue when it came to what aims should drive breeding, it was not the only one. In the next chapter, reasons for a breeding emphasis on certain colours will be examined. It will be clear that beauty or interest in fancy was often not a dictator in specialization for colour.

Chapter Five

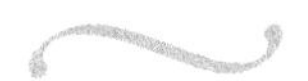

Implications of Breeding for Colour

One major aspect driving selection aims relates to specialization for colour, and, like all other breeding aims, the favouring of certain colours presents a many-sided story. Regulation of accepted colours in breeds has played a significant role in the production of many animals, particularly members of the purebred breeds. Purebred cattle, horse, and dog breeds all have colour restrictions. For example, Angus cattle that are black cannot have more than a few patches of white, and these must be located on the underbelly. Only recently could Angus be red. Shorthorns can never be black. Holsteins had to be black and white, not red and white, until the 1980s. Hereford cattle were deliberately bred to preserve and emphasize the white face – all other colours were avoided. It was believed that the white face made Herefords a recognizable "brand." Certain horse breeds are defined solely on the basis of colour, the Palomino and Pinto being examples. Many dog breeds have colour regulations set out in the standards which govern their purebred status. Beauty or interest in fancy was, however, by no means the only driver in breeding for colour. Various colour-breeding situations assessed in this chapter make it evident that the motivation to select for colour arose from complicated and differing factors.

Breeding as a Sport: Barred Plymouth Rocks and Colour

Selection for colour over the late nineteenth and early twentieth century in the North American standardbred chicken world seemed in some cases to be driven more by what could be called sport of breeding than colour concerns. Continuing regulations on what defined beauty in colour for the Barred Plymouth Rock seemed to go hand in hand with breeder interest in assessing levels of breeding skill. Colour, under these conditions, was intended to provide visual proof of a person's ability to breed. Because the Barred Plymouth Rock played a central role in the utility poultry industry, it is worth starting this discussion about the sport of breeding and colour by looking briefly at the bird's background and characteristics.[1]

Americans had created the Barred Plymouth Rock between roughly 1864 and 1875 by crossbreeding a number of different types, then inbreeding certain lines to make the bird breed truly, but always balancing that inbreeding with the outcross breeding of unrelated families to avoid inbreeding weakness. The result was a useful bird, even if early lines did not always produce consistent results as to type. Dual purpose, the Barred Rocks incubated their eggs: they were "sitters," unlike the breed that in the end came to dominate the egg industry, the Leghorn. Vigorous, active, and with a foraging instinct, the Rocks were also relatively heavy, making them good meat birds, also unlike the Leghorn. Because the Rocks provided both meat and eggs, incubated their eggs, and were able to fend for themselves naturally, they quickly became favourites of women producers in the United States and Canada.[2] (The history and use of the Rock, then, provides an example of how important a dual purpose was with feminine production. The Leghorn would come to dominate the table egg industry only when masculine control and emphasis on single purpose had evolved.)

Colour became a particularly important feature in beauty ideology as applied to Barred Rocks when standards set by the American Poultry Association for the breed demanded that male and female be identical in colour depth and shape of barring (or stripes) across the bird's body and wings. Females, however, had a tendency to be darker than the males, owing to the sex inheritance mechanism of colour and the barring trait. Trying to make the birds of both sexes match a single standard, then, was tricky and in the end supported the idea that breeding could be pursued simply as a sport. A method known as double mating quickly arose and was designed to overcome the colour difficulty inherent in the way standards for Rocks had been laid out. The method first appeared in Britain.[3]

The double mating system called for breeding of one line for producing good males and one for good females, therefore not for efforts at getting the correct males and females from one mating. The two lines were to be created in the following manner: one by mating females producing especially good hens to males producing particularly good hens, and the other by mating females producing good males to males producing good males. For the production of correctly coloured hens, breeders were advised to select females of the perfect colour and breed males to them that were lighter in normal male colour and therefore not of desirable colour. But while the male should be lighter than his mate, his barring should be as perfect as possible. When high-class females had been obtained year after year from such matings, the males that resulted in such breedings, while not perfect from a colour point of view, would be invaluable as hen producers. To breed correctly coloured final males, breeders should select large females in shades considerably darker than was considered correct and put these dark females to perfectly coloured males. The resulting females would not be of good colour, but they could be useful for the production of perfectly coloured males.[4] The emphasis on deep barring marks – in fact through the feathers and down to the skin – increased the need for double mating. The only way to achieve identical and proper colour in both male and female was to breed within a double mating system. Colour, of course, was just one consideration. Size, shape, and other qualities were selected for as well, making such a breeding program demanding.[5] (The culls from these breeding exercises would be commercially used by women producers.)

The correct males and females from this breeding program, then, were useless as breeding pairs for show stock, thereby creating a sort of biological lock. The breeding lines produced the "best," but members of one sex in each line were not the "best" in themselves. The practice of keeping two lines to achieve correct colour annoyed many Barred Plymouth Rock fanciers who not only saw the breeding method as cumbersome and unnecessarily difficult but also argued that male and female Barred Rocks were designed by nature to be a different colour.[6] It was simply going against nature to set up beauty standards that were so incompatible with hereditary laws. Some believed that, over time and with careful selection, males and females would be brought closer together in barring characteristics and in underlying colour within one line (but this had not been accomplished by the 1920s, and by then most had come to accept the fact that barring was sex-linked).[7]

Many argued that since the Barred Rock naturally threw a variation in colour due to its hereditary background, an overemphasis on colour led to a sacrifice of good overall shape.[8] Others, however, avoided discussion around the colour standards problem because they recognized that the double mating system in fact had never really been about valuing colour as such in the first place. They emphasized that the double mating system held worth, not so much because of its power to create properly coloured birds of both sexes, but rather because it taught skill. The difficulty of breeding by the method was, in fact, what made it so important. It tested a breeder's mettle. The method drew the best breeders to the Barred Rock, breeders who wanted to learn more about the skill of breeding.[9] It was lessons in breeding, not so much the results of breeding or even colour itself, that made the double mating system valuable.

Breeding of the Barred Plymouth Rock for designated correct colour reveals interesting patterns; perhaps most significantly why attitudes to fancy could lead to standards that demanded the use of such a complex system. Breeders adhered to this standard, admired more for its testing of skill than its ability to bring about more useful birds, and resisted any efforts at revising it. The challenge behind breeding for sport was in this case to create an "unnatural" colour. There seemed to be little reason for setting beauty standards which went against natural inheritance patterns of colour, other than facing a difficult challenge. The existence of two standards – one for male and one for female – would mean the end of the double mating system and allowed for easier ways of breeding the birds. The fact that sufficient support within the Barred Rock world for such a move did not occur tends to confirm the reality that the sport of breeding was the driver for maintaining the single colour standard.

Industry Requirements: Cattle Breeding and Colour

Breeding as a sport, with colour characteristics as its object, was one factor in colour selection. Industry requirements proved to be another. Attitudes to white Shorthorn cattle in the late nineteenth century serve as a significant example of that pattern. One particular animal, a high-quality Shorthorn male, can effectively introduce this review of how such a chain of events reflecting industry requirements could evolve. The night this Shorthorn was born in Ontario, a cold and clear one in February 1881, he aroused great disappointment in the people around him. When going out to see "this unwelcome arrival," the men stood dejectedly beside the newborn calf's stall, just as the baby was "getting up on his forelegs seeking for food. He was a lusty chap and white as the snow outside." Because of his whiteness, the calf, Clarence Kirklevington, became a steer and not a breeding bull, in spite of the fact that his future career in the ring would demonstrate his excellence. Three years after his birth, that is in 1884, Clarence won every class possible in Chicago, the centre of North America's beef cattle industry. He was champion Shorthorn steer of any age, the best animal of any breed, and ultimately the best carcass of any breed or age.[10] The fact that white Clarence lived at the height of the red craze for Shorthorns dictated his future. The American fad for the red colour clearly meant that a potentially top quality bull of any other colour would be lost for breeding purposes, a situation which suggested a worrying trend as far as many cattlemen at the time were concerned.

It certainly puzzled many Canadians because of its evident nonsensical basis, as the 1880 conversation that introduced this book makes clear. The issue provoked much discussion everywhere in agricultural circles, especially when it seemed likely that the emphasis on breeding for red would lead to a considerable number of inferior animals. William Brown, professor at the Ontario Agricultural College, remarked on the American avoidance of white as early as 1878.

> I have failed to get one sound reason for the prejudice that at present exists against white cattle, especially in America ... There can be no objection to a fashion in colours, by the taste of the breeder, or in those who purchase; but we must have *facts* for any inferiority. It is well known that most of the eminent short-horn progenitors were pure white, and looking at the prize rings in Britain now, it will be found that white still takes off most of the honours.[11]

In 1886, the *Canadian Live-Stock and Farm Journal* printed an article called "The Red, White and Roan – Which Color Should We Adopt?" which concluded that the red colour craze was confined to the United States, but that if Ontario breeders wanted that market, they had better breed more reds.[12] The *Farmer's Advocate,* in an article called "Color in Shorthorns," reported in 1909 on recent sales of Shorthorns: solid red was still preferred by buyers who were American Shorthorn breeders. Canadian breeders, as a result, were prepared to breed for red, and that trend showed the strength of the almighty dollar, because red was known to be the worst colour for Shorthorns.[13] An important Ontario breeder agreed, saying: "Dark red ruined Cattle in the U.S. ... what now is Called [*sic*] the *Colour Craze.* Dark red was always unpopular in Scotland ... [Red Shorthorns] have the worst hair & the thinnest flesh."[14] Another stated that he "never knew any man who could breed Shorthorns unless he bred some white ones."[15] But quality had no effect on purebred market values. The *Canadian Live-Stock and Farm Journal* claimed that a red bull would sell in Chicago no matter what his quality was.[16] By 1885 white bulls could not be sold even to commercial, or non-purebred, breeders.[17] One Ontario breeder, T. Russell, found he could not sell any of his stock because there were reports of white Shorthorns in his herd. Another offered to replace a good white bull calf with a red heifer for a buyer in Wisconsin.[18] The American rejection of white and the concurrent demand for red influenced important breeders in Scotland who exported stock to Canadian importers, Amos Cruickshank being one.[19]

American breeders were just as disenchanted by the new demand for red as their Canadian counterparts. While they railed against it, however, they understood aspects of the basis for the demand better than did the Canadians. A former president of the American Shorthorn Association, T.C. Jones, wrote a thoughtful letter in 1881 to the *Breeder's Gazette* about the issue. He addressed the well-known desire of Western ranchmen for red bulls and the "nonsense contained in letters sometimes written from the West for the instruction of Short-Horn breeders in regard to the taste of the ranchmen in Texas and the Territories. We are advised that we must breed red bulls; nothing else will suit; they must be all red … or the ranchmen will not buy them." Western agents were sent to buy such stock. But, Jones argued, the Western preference for red was in reality only a fashion because it was not based on reason. One rancher's views served Jones as an example of the irrationality of wanting only red. "Give me a red Short-Horn bull in preference to anything else for a Texan or Mexican cow," the man told Jones, who responded by asking why. "Because I like them" was the answer. Jones pointed out the absurdity, rationally speaking, of such reasoning. Apparently at least some ranchmen had no logical basis for demanding red, as far as Jones was concerned.[20] Jones considered breeding simply for red an ill-advised strategy. It had nothing to do with either quality or improvement.

Other breeders supported this view. "For if there ever was a foolish craze, this red mania is certainly one. Being a small breeder I have felt almost compelled to breed such as the general buyer wanted, which is contrary to both my taste and my Judgement," wrote Newton Frazier to the *Gazette*.[21] T.C. Anderson, in a letter to the *Gazette* entitled "Red Short-Horns," put the issue more strongly. "I have not a doubt in my mind that this thing of selecting a [red] bull to head Short-Horn herds has worked more harm to those herds than all other causes combined. If it be a fashion, how it got started is quite a wonder to me."[22] Jones and others might have understood the demands of cow/calf operators to be somewhat irrational, but they did not grasp the fact that while some cow/calf operators seemed to be simply following what had become an established trend, other members of that group had set that trend because they had found that calves from red bulls suited the feeder market better than mixed coloured calves. Fundamentally what Shorthorn breeders really railed against was the power of the market linkage from purebred breeder to cow/calf operator to feeder sector. All branches were subject to the demands of the others, whether considered desirable or not. That meant that Western rancher demands could infect purebred breeder aims.

Changing trends within the complicated structure of the North American beef industry were behind the demand for red. An emphasis on red began on the Western range of the United States, where ranchers, fundamentally cow/calf operators, preferred solid coloured and dark red Shorthorn bulls to cross on Texas Longhorn females. Ranchers had found that the use of whites and roans resulted in strangely coloured calves which were hard to sell to feeder operations. That situation forced the ranchers to breed for feeder stock using red bulls, which consequently made their bull suppliers, Shorthorn breeders in the Midwest and through them some Ontario breeders as well, select for red. Purebred breeders in the Midwest acquiesced by breeding red Shorthorns and avoiding white or roan and even light coloured red. (Canadians increasingly would follow suit.) As Alvin Sanders, editor of the *Breeder's Gazette*, explained:

> The buyers of bulls for steer-getting purposes were inexorable. A solid red, and worst of all (in many cases) very dark red bulls, of the most ordinary character, were freely bought in preference to thicker, better, mellower roans, yellow-reds or reds with white markings. So general was this demand at one time that it seemed fairly suicidal for the owners of pedigreed herds to use any other than red bulls. The pursuit of this policy led to the sacrifice of many useful cattle.[23]

In 1936, after the demand for red had passed, Sanders elaborated on the red craze of the late nineteenth century as follows:

> Not only were the roan and white bulls discredited, and in many cases discarded entirely, by those who depended upon the big Western market for the surplus bulls of the Corn Belt states, but the consequent limitation of the choice of color in herd bulls to the solid reds led inevitably to the use of many bulls in Mid-West herds that were really sub-standard, so far as substance and general confirmation was concerned. Color, in other words, was the paramount consideration in selecting stock bulls. That this had a deteriorating influence upon the breed, as a whole, in the States was obvious; and the tendency towards a lower standard of individual merit operated to contribute to the ready welcome accorded the Herefords and Aberdeen-Angus upon their first introduction into America. Fortunately, when the peak of the Western demand for red bulls had passed, pressure upon the score of color was happily removed from those who raced the competition of the "white-faces" and the blacks.[24]

All Shorthorn cattle were, in fact, roan coloured, and when the Colour Craze broke out, misunderstandings of that fact did not help the situation. One of the first issues that breeders interested in genetics hoped the new science would solve was the way colour patterns worked in Shorthorns. As Dryden said to fellow Ontario breeders in 1904, "there are problems we don't understand. A red sire and rich roan dam produce a white calf. How does it come? Who can answer? Yet I have a firm conviction that [it is] controlled by some (to us) unknown law."[25] It would be the science of genetics and its understanding of the genes controlling roaning that would solve the puzzle of Shorthorn colouring. An early genetic breakthrough with respect to livestock production came in the 1920s with a better understanding of roaning.[26] Roan is a colour made by the diffusion of red and white pigmentation. What is significant about that diffusion, however, is that the overall colour effect of the animal is achieved through an intermingling of purely red and purely white individual hairs throughout the coat.[27] Individual animals carried different percentages of red and white hairs. Cattle varied, then, from what appeared to be solid red to solid white. In reality, all had at least a small proportion of both red and white hairs, even though individuals could be almost deficient in either. Red Shorthorns were merely roans with an overwhelming number of red hairs. White Shorthorns were merely roans with an overwhelming number of white hairs. "Roan" Shorthorns were roans with a more equal number of red and white hairs. When roaning became better understood after the 1920s, white Shorthorns became popular, and some amateurs deliberately kept herds that were purely white.

Knowledge of the genetic base for roaning and its relationship to red probably helped defuse rancher demand for red because of a change of feeder farmer views. However, it is possible that the shifts in rancher and feeder operator attitudes to red merely occurred simultaneously with the rise of new genetic knowledge. The rising popularity of the solid or uniform colouration of the Angus and Hereford breeds probably played a more important role in defusing the desire for only red Shorthorns. The move away from obsession with red, however, allowed Shorthorn breeders to breed for quality and subsequently to hold their markets in the West after Angus and Herefords began to offer competition. As Sanders said, it became possible to breed for better Shorthorns, not just red Shorthorns. Shorthorn breeders everywhere had seen the pressure to select for red as detrimental to the breed, because they associated dark red with inferior animals.

Canadian breeders persisted throughout the time of the craze and after its passage in seeing the breeding for red as an American purebred fad and a fancy. Midwest breeders in the United States had tended to agree, but since the cow/calf operator market for their bulls dictated that red was in demand to the exclusion of any other colour, for these breeders it was primarily a trade issue. Nothing could more forcefully show the linkage of the beef cattle industry sectors: the dependence of purebred breeders on cow/calf operator demand, and ultimately the wants of the feeder (producer) arm. Ontario breeders, in particular, never came to see how forceful that complicated market had been in driving purebred breeding patterns, perhaps because they did not appreciate how significant the complicated chain leading back to cow/calf operators on the American rangeland in conjunction with feeder operators closer to the Midwest actually was or how, ultimately, that situation affected their breeding work in Canada. For Shorthorn breeders in Ontario, breeding for red was just another American fad, but a fad that they, as breeders, had to deal with if they wanted to sell cattle in the United States. The "almighty dollar," as they called it, made breeders respond to a fancy market as well as a commercial beef market.

Industry Requirements: The Breeding of Hybrid, Egg-Laying Chickens and Colour

One might think that the revolution which ended the control of the beauty breeding base of the chicken industry, which came with the rise of hybrid breeding for utility by the 1940s, would end any emphasis on selection for colour. That, however, would not be the case. The fate of the Barred Plymouth Rock and other chicken breeds in the hybrid breeding chicken world of the mid-twentieth century would match that of white Shorthorns in the late nineteenth century, again because of industry requirements. Consumer demand dictated which chickens would serve the table egg industry. All breeding had to reflect consumer preference for certain colour in eggs, regardless of which hybrid hens could be made to be the most superior producers. Nothing could more conclusively prove that fancy (at least fancy as dictated by breeder aesthetics) was often not the most important factor driving selection by colour. When breeding for table eggs began to be more commercially significant in North America, four breeds had proven they could excel in that department: the Leghorn, the Plymouth Rock (Barred or White), the Wyandotte, and the Rhode Island Red. The fate of these breeds in the egg industry – which breed would get the most attention under the hybrid breeding systems – would rest on consumer preference by region for egg colour. The Leghorn produce white eggs, the Rocks, Rhode Island Red, and Wyandotte produce brown eggs. This fact alone, not level of production, drove which breed the breeding companies would work with. North Americans preferred white eggs (New England was the only major centre in North America which favoured brown eggs); therefore Leghorns would dominate the North American egg industry.

The overwhelming popularity of white eggs with consumers in North America enforced not only an emphasis on Leghorns when breeding companies undertook hybrid breeding in the 1930s but also the avoidance of synthetic lines on the basis of various breed compositions. The challenge of creating such lines variable enough to produce hybrid vigour when crossed was, therefore, more difficult. Fortunately for the breeding companies, the Leghorn was unusual in that it could be bred to result in many strains divergent from each other, thereby creating "breeds" of true lines within a single breed. Leghorns responded well to selection for distinct lines within the one breed. It was assumed that the reason for this was that the Leghorn carried a smaller genetic load, meaning it had fewer potential lethal recessives that could surface in a homozygous state than did the Rocks and other breeds established in the late nineteenth century in North America.[28] Perhaps the antiquity of the Leghorn breed, going back to Roman times, played a role in that freedom from defective recessives. They had been largely eliminated through selection centuries ago. Introduced to North America in 1828 from Italy, the modern Leghorn was developed in the United States through crossing with white Minorcas and further importation from Italy in 1840 and 1845.[29]

The Leghorn would not dominate the egg-breeding industry in Europe because Europeans preferred brown eggs. Breeding companies could not use the Leghorn in crossbreeding programs either, because crosses with brown egg breeds often resulted in eggs coloured somewhere in between and described as "tinted" eggs. These were not desirable in any widespread way. But crossbreeding could be used as a strategy by the companies if they stayed with the brown egg laying breeds. By 2007 it was estimated that the commercial brown egg hen came mainly from a Rhode Island Red male and a White Plymouth Rock female. Smaller brown eggs resulted from a reversed sex cross of these two.[30] The birds served a market in England, France, Belgium, Italy, and Portugal, where brown eggs sold at a rate of 98 to 100 per cent versus white. Spain's market was about 50 per cent each. (In North America the market share of brown eggs to total was only 5 per cent by the 1980s.)[31]

Genetics versus Aesthetics: Collie (or Lassie Type) Breeding and Colour

A review of North American and British attitudes to one colour in a purebred dog breed, namely white in Collies (or Lassie type dogs), reveals the complexity of the motivational issues driving breeding for colour.[32] Attitudes to white in Collies, when looked at as they evolved over time, also show that breeding convictions with respect to colour could endure for centuries. The white Collie story makes it clear that entrenched traditional perceptions concerning heredity remained in force, in spite of advancements in science; and shows as well that views on what defined beauty were irrevocably tied up with non-aesthetic ideas.[33] Historically, North American and British breeders held different views concerning white, a critical fact behind this story as it evolved across two centuries. American and Canadian Collie breeders always considered predominantly white coats to be a mark of beauty, while British breeders persisted in seeing white coats as undesirable. This differing attitude towards coat colour was laid down between 1890 and 1920, and looking at how that situation arose does much to explain aspects of apparent breeding for fancy. The story also introduces a larger topic: how can breeding practices, based on complicated historical perceptions that arose from a beauty versus science axis, be altered to reflect modern ethical concerns?

The dominant original colours for "colleys" in Britain had been black or a grey-blue colour known as blue merle. White markings with blue merle or black had not been desired.[34] With the evolution of the new dog fancy, though, markets could be sensitive to colour style, and breeders responded to that situation by changing the varieties available in Collies. Black with tan markings became popular by the late 1860s. Collies of this colour found a ready market, even if some serious breeders believed the dogs to be mongrels – crosses between Collies and Gordon Setters. One early Collie expert described the new trend as resulting in dogs with "thin coats 'soft as a lady's hand', feathered legs, draggle tails, saddle-flap ears, and a rich mahogany-color kissing spot on each cheek."[35] The introduction of the colour sable in the 1870s – gold to mahogany – would be crucial to the subsequent welfare of all Collie colours. First, it reduced the popularity of blue merle and of black and tan. More significantly, however, sable made white in the form of markings desirable. The presence of white with sable became popular and led to white markings being combined with any of the other Collie colours.

This trend towards white markings went against historic Collie breeding and was not without difficulty. Whiteness had traditionally been problematic for early British breeders, because of their experience with all-white dogs arising from merle to merle matings. Even if they did not understand the effects of the gene that created the blue-grey colour, that is the merling gene, British breeders had long known that merle to merle crosses could result in pure white Collies, but the dogs were often defective as well. Breeders learned to link whiteness with inherent unsoundness, because experience taught them that white dogs could be blind, deaf, or weak. Most white puppies had been killed at birth – farmers believing them to be what would today be described as genetic misfits.[36] The rise of sable and white made white markings acceptable, but all-white was another matter.

The flowering of the Collie fancy and the growing trend towards creating more colours made a few breeders in Britain decide to concentrate on breeding for pure white or nearly pure white dogs in spite of the dangers that some would be defective.[37] John Storey of Scotland bred exclusively for white. He was clever in marketing his breeding: he allied himself with Queen Victoria's dog interests.[38] Victoria's love of dogs was legendary, and she housed and enjoyed many at her Windsor kennels.[39] She had been presented with a white Collie by the Earl of Haddington and soon became so enamoured with white in Collies that allegedly she offered a thousand pounds for anyone who could deliver a pure white Collie to Windsor. In 1882 the queen made a trip to Edinburgh, and Storey had his four dogs stationed on a raised platform so that she could see them on her way.[40] The concern of a few breeders for white dogs, however, did not grow into a widespread movement. By 1900, all-white dogs in Britain were again avoided, as breeders returned to the long-held view that the colour was undesirable in Collies because of its linkage to poor quality (aka defective characteristics).

All-white Collies became popular in the United States at the end of the nineteenth century, when interest in them had evaporated in Britain. These white dogs resulted from an emphasis on the gene that produced white markings, a gene prevalent in Collie DNA since the advent of sable and white in the 1870s. With the white marking gene, it was possible to create nearly pure white dogs that were not likely to be defective because their whiteness had nothing to do with the merling gene. "The fad for white Collies has been alive for a number of years now," *Country Life in America* noted in 1915. White Collies were bred from sable and white dogs with a great deal of white, the journal said, and the crossing of all-white pups from sable and white parents has resulted in "the running back for seven or eight generations of all-white collies."

A breeder explained how the true variety of white Collie came into existence in the United States. "The white collie was originally a sport [i.e., a fluke] from a whelping of pups of the sable collie. Breeders of sable collies in past years have been trying to breed an extra heavy white collar, and in doing so they have inbred to a certain extent, so that all-white sports [flukes] have occasionally been produced from the breeding. These all-white pups, from different litters, have been crossed and recrossed, so that to-day the white collie is a standard variety."[41] One breeder, Fred Avery, made it a business to produce white Collie pups for the pet market, and he could turn out 100 puppies (not necessarily all of which were white) a month by farming out at least 350 bitches to trusted neighbours.[42] A 1916 ad in *Country Life in America* for the Island White Collie Kennels in Wisconsin stated, "A white Scotch Collie has no equal ... White Scotch Collies embody all dog virtues."[43] The popularity of white dogs reached a peak between 1920 and 1925.[44] The Collie Club of America set up a committee in 1925 to look into how to judge a white Collie. No conclusion was reached.[45]

The persistent selection for the colour white with little regard for other or more desirable points for show purposes by American breeders (and possibly the interbreeding with white Samoyeds)[46] resulted in a type of all-white Collie that was not of top quality from an exhibition point of view, and did not look like the purebred Collie being produced by 1900. The trend towards non-modern Collies escalated into the 1920s.[47] Pictures of them in articles on all-white Collies reveal that many presented a true reversion to the older style found in the early Scottish sheepdogs or "colleys": heavy heads, low ears, and short bushy coats. The dogs commanded no respect from serious breeders who were trying to achieve a form of beauty that could successfully compete in the Kennel Club shows. Collie experts in both the United States and Britain dismissed the American white Collie as a fad for a fancy type of pet. The reintroduction of interest in the blue merle colour led to a crystallization of attitudes towards all-white in both Britain and the United States, and laid down the groundwork for a growing cultural cleavage between the two countries in relation to the evaluation of pure white.

Shortly after the turn of the century, a reaction to the predominant sable colour set in and triggered a desire in Britain to breed more blue merles, a colour that had all but disappeared. The British *Collie Folio* devoted a separate section to the breeding of blue merles. This would be the only colour for which the journal provided space to pursue matters pertaining specifically to the issue of colour. The much more dominant sables had no such section devoted to them, earlier or later, from a colour point of view. New attempts to select for the blue merle colour led, naturally, to the increased breeding of blue merle to blue merle in Britain, a practice that produces some defective white dogs, and by 1910 defective whites were not uncommon in puppy litters resulting from this breeding strategy. In the early twentieth century, then, two different types of white Collies were being produced: double merles in Britain and dominant white from the marking gene in the United States.

Marketability seemed to repress any desire to understand the biological issues that created white in Collies. While early breeders were not privy to knowledge about how genes work, distinguishing which breeding selections would likely lead to lethal or benign white was certainly within their power. British breeders either could not or would not recognize that white Collies derived from sables, blacks, or tricolours (black, tan, and white) were not the same as white Collies derived from merle to merle breeding, and that genetic soundness was a dividing question between the two. Did defectiveness in a biological product not matter when the buyer had already demonstrated a lack of appreciation for quality with respect to fancy points? Did marketability cancel the need to know what caused white and what caused problems in some whites and not in others? White, after all, was white, and since all whites were of poor quality aesthetically, why did it matter that one type was known to show inferiority by being fundamentally unsound as well? It would appear that some British breeders were prepared to breed and export double merle whites in order to supply Americans with white dogs.

The *Collie Folio* advised British breeders to save these white rejects and export them to the United States. "It seems possible that Merle breeders in England who at times get these 'misfits' as a result of too closely following colour lines, ought to put themselves in touch with buyers through our columns. Better to spend a few dollars in this way than to bucket the unwelcome ones." "There is no accounting for taste, but it would appear to be bad business to drown puppies in England which are wanted in America," the journal added.[48] William Mason, editor of the *Folio* and an astute Collie breeder and marketer, chose not to distinguish American whites, unattractive as they may have been to him, from defective whites. The poor show quality of the popular white Collie in the United States, the influx of double merles from Britain, and the subsequent American breeding of merle to merle for all-white dogs[49] made breeders in the United States more aware of the defective white problem. By 1930 all-white dogs had lost popularity, tinged now with the double merle spectre. Sound white Collies, the results of the marking gene, would not gain even minimal respectability in Collie breeding and exhibition ranks until the late 1930s, after Americans began to select for dogs that were not pure white (it would be Fred Avery who started that process in the 1920s), but rather had coloured heads.[50]

The decline of the white Collie in the United States, however, did not mean white dogs vanished from the scene. The culture laid down in that country from 1890 to 1910 was resilient enough to keep the breeding of these dogs alive, and strengthened the desire to separate double merle breeding of whites from the more traditional American method of breeding them; namely emphasizing excessive white markings. Various white Collie associations were founded and failed, the first being in 1949. (A surviving association, under the name of the International White Collie Club, was not founded until 2000.)[51] In spite of the fact that white Collies continued to be exhibited in the United States, it would not be until 1950 that American Collie breeders agreed to change their written standard, the American Collie Standard, and accept white as a recognized colour.[52] Even so, merle coloured heads on white dogs were not recognized until the Standard's revision in 1977.[53] Residual fears concerning the role of double merling in the predominantly white coat remained, even though by that time the colour genetics of dogs was clearly understood.

The subject had attracted considerable interest from scientists over the years. They were actively studying how inheritance of merling worked by the 1930s.[54] C.C. Little wrote his classic work on dog genetics in 1957, proving that separate genes governed whiteness in Collies and explaining how merling played a role in one form of whiteness.[55] He showed that whiteness can result from the effects of three separate genes. The genes, acting in a variety of ways when paired differently through inheritance, result in predominantly white Collies: C or the albino series, which prohibits colour; S or the spotting gene series, which provides the white ruff collar and other white markings on Collies, and can deliver whiteness so excessively that it virtually extends over all the body; and M or the merling gene, which produces white when two copies of the M allele are inherited.[56] Benign predominant whiteness is most likely to occur through the spotting gene series, but all three genetic factors can result in defects, generally relating to hearing and seeing. Double merling (MM) is the most lethal in this respect.

The merling gene dilutes colour; it is not a colour in itself. Neither is merling related to albinism, which causes absence of colour, not dilution. Merling weakens colour (in double merles it weakens colour almost out of existence), while albinism blocks all colour expression. Albinism is also a recessive trait, while merling is an incomplete dominant trait. Blue merles are dogs that carry one copy of the merle allele (M) that represses what would have been black in coat colour. A dog with one copy of the M allele has the genotype Mm (heterozygous merle). If a dog carries two M alleles, having a genotype of MM (homozygous merle or double merle), which can happen in a merle to merle mating, it will end up being white: the black is diluted to such a degree that there is effectively little or no colour in the dog's coat. A double M allele dog is known as a defective white, because the merle allele, when doubled, also affects internal pigment necessary for the development of nerve fibres associated with seeing and hearing. Defective whites often, as a result, are blind and deaf, and many do not survive birth.[57] The gene responsible for merling was located in DNA in 2006.[58]

Opening the door in 1950 to the acceptability of white coloured coats carried with it official recognition of double merles via pedigreeing, and therefore their presence in the breeding pool. Double merles continued to be bred in the United States throughout the twentieth and into the twenty-first century, and there is some evidence that the breeding of double merles even increased over that period.[59] Their very existence, let alone presence in the show ring under the classification of white, fuelled underlying suspicions concerning quality in dogs that were all-white from the spotting gene.[60] More problematic, however, was the use of double merles to generate guaranteed merles: a double merle is almost certain to produce only merle puppies.

A controversy arose in 2012 when a merle Collie, sired by a double merle, won Best of Breed at the Westminster Dog Show. Chat lines on the Internet showed general outrage at this form of breeding. Of particular significance was the chat line called "Border Wars" and run by Christopher Laudauer, a lover of Border Collies.[61] Discussion on the Internet over the issue was hot and lengthy. Finally Collie breeders felt called to respond. An article appeared in the March 2012 edition of the *American Kennel Club Gazette*. "The ability to critically evaluate where we are in confirmation, temperament, and health issues is essential to the future of dog breeding in general and our breed specifically," wrote Marianne Sullivan.[62] She elaborated as follows:

> Moral and ethical questions evolve with the times, but shouldn't common sense tell us that breeding dogs who can't … see or hear is wrong? Aside from the breeder's perspective, what about the person willing to take a blind or deaf dog, or even the dog's point of view? The argument that these dogs live good, happy lives ignores the fact that they are still unnecessarily handicapped and have a compromised life … Public perception will not go away, and it is time for us to start taking control of the message.

> If we don't behave consistently and clearly as though the health of our dogs is of primary importance, there are those who will take control of the message for us.[63]

The double merle versus blue merle issue became entangled in the United States with what is known as the sable merle. Merling can effect sable coloured dogs the same way that black coats are affected, namely by dilution. It is here that a hidden menace from double merling was believed to present itself. Sable merles can be hard to recognize without DNA testing (which can be done), and therefore double merling could unintentionally result from an unknown sable merle bred to a known blue merle. Many American breeders today love the softened gold colour of sable merles, and over the years various campaigns have been launched to separate the sable merle from the sable, thereby making the sable merle acceptable in its own right, in the same way that the white or blue merle is. The last effort took place over 2008 and 2009, stimulating much discussion on the Internet. A Standards Committee of the Collie Club of America, which assessed any revisions or amendments to the Collie standard, looked into the issue in 2009 but did not recommend changing it to establish the sable merle. Sable merles continue to be unrecognized as a separate colour in the written standard, in spite of the fact that they are just as sound as blue merles. Cultural attitudes towards white laid down between 1890 and 1910 in the United States would dictate a continuing interest in all-white Collies, but brought with it a myriad of problems. White might arise from different selection methods which were founded on varying DNA sources, but clarification of that fact never seemed to take hold. The spectre of double merling dogged the fortunes of blue merles for a considerable length of time, fuelled the conflict surrounding sable merles, and continues to flavour many views about any all-white dogs. Only the sable and the tricolour have remained free of the curse, culturally speaking, of the merling gene. Perceiving all-white to be a mark of beauty apparently did not come without price.

Double merling has not inflamed conflicts in British breeding of Collies in a similar fashion because all-white, as a result of the spotting gene, has never been accepted in the United Kingdom. The spectre of double merling made British breeders resist white from the benign spotting gene, and consequently shaped their views on the aesthetic value of the white coat. In fact, avoidance of excessive white outside the United States has resulted in a much-reduced gene pool of dogs carrying the normal gene for white in most other countries.[64] Attitudes towards the desirability of all-white, laid down for centuries as a result of the old merle to merle breeding, remain in place and reflect cultural inclinations as much as understanding of genetics.[65] Collie colours accepted today under the British Collie Standard are sable and white, tricolour, and blue merle and white. Neither all-white nor sable merles are recognized. Prejudice against these colours, evident in breed standards which reject all-whites and sable merles, might have evolved originally from the desire to restrict the production of double merles, but today they are as much about aesthetics as genetics.

More rigorous action to prohibit double merle breeding emerged in Europe before it did in Britain, via the European Convention for the Protection of Pet Animals (Council of Europe Treaty Series 125) established in 1987.[66] In 1995 the Convention strengthened its Article 5, which was designed to control breeding practices that were detrimental to canine health, by offering specific examples of matings to be avoided. (The Federation Cynologique Internationale or FCI – a body that affects dog breeders in many European countries – takes a similar stand on the matter.)[67] One suggestion was to prohibit breeding of any merle animals from any canine breed where the merling colour existed, let alone double merles. Britain was not a signatory of the Convention, but in 2006 it decided to revisit the problem of unethical breeding. By 2009 there was mounting pressure in that country from various organizations to put in place regulations to control how breeding of British dogs proceeded.[68] In 2012 the Kennel Club announced that, as of January 2013, it would no longer pedigree puppies of any breed resulting from any merle to merle breeding.[69] Since these dogs could no longer be registered, the value in producing double merles from such matings evaporated under the purebred system. They could not be used for breeding. Regulation to control the production of double merles had gone beyond colour recognition of breeders.

The linkage of white with double merling and the defects that often accompany double merling has affected the breeding of many Collie coat colours across nations (only sable and tricolour escaped contamination), but not always in logical ways that reflect an appreciation of how genetics works – at least not under breed standards set by specialty clubs. Preconceived ideas about what makes quality and what makes beauty are evidently clearly resistant to change within certain circles of the dog-breeding world. The difference in situation between North America and Britain implies that outside pressure can result in reorientation to such issues under certain conditions. The regulation in place today in Britain, with regard to the actual breeding of double merles, indicates a greater willingness than can be found in North America to bow to outside pressure. Britain's stance resembles, even if it does not actually mirror, the situation on the Continent, where state-enforced control is more evident. The fact that Collie breeders in both Britain and Europe do not like white as a dominant colour made the reform easier. General acceptance of white as a mark of beauty by North American Collie breeders (and recognition as such in their breed standards) helps to reinforce the continuation of double merle pedigreeing by US kennel clubs. The connection of genetic understanding with colour inheritance was clearly a factor in both Barred Plymouth Rock and Collie breeding. Even when the issue of colour was fancy-oriented or at least not utility-oriented, genetics and the understanding of genetic laws at any given point in time have influenced attitudes and concurrently what colours defined beauty.

But another factor plays a role in this story; namely the breeders' belief that they should have the liberty to breed as they wish without outside interference, thereby ensuring their strong resistance to any pressure for change exerted by either kennel clubs or other organizations. Outside control over breeder strategies through various government structures has for some time been far stricter in Europe, and effectively in Britain as well, than in either the United States or Canada. The force with which breeder organizations in North America cling to what they believe are their rights has arguably fed into the growth of ever more virulent animal welfare and rights organizations attempting to control breeder activity. The North American breeder stance that they are at liberty to breed as they see fit may become an increasingly difficult position to hold in light of modern ethical concerns. Marianne Sullivan's words seem prophetic.

Chapter Six

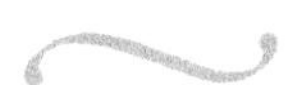

Breeding for Authenticity

I noted in the first section of this book that environmental breeding and its tenets never completely disappeared with the rise of improvement breeding. But it is also true that the idea of improving was not entirely new at that time. Environmental and improvement breeding concepts have always been entangled with each other, at least to some degree. In this chapter I show that it is important to recognize that entanglement because, by doing so, characteristics of a major twentieth-century breeding movement, that is authenticity breeding, make more sense. I begin by providing examples of the ongoing entanglement. I look first at improvement breeding in the era of environmental breeding, and then at environmental breeding during the era of improvement breeding. It will be apparent that under both conditions, whatever the desired result, meticulous selection characterized all breeding. It was never random selection. The point is well worth making and goes a long way in pointing out the existence of fundamental similarities between environmental and improvement breeding.

Efforts at improvement breeding can be seen in the different ways that two seventeenth-century horse breeders in England worked with a geohumour theory, important to breeders at the time. The geohumour theory postulated that the four standard humours (established by Aristotle) could be understood as aspects of the climate. The climate-based humours were hot and dry, dry and cold, cold and moist, and moist and hot. Resting on the theory of opposites as set out by Galen (a Greek thinker who developed various medical hypotheses in the second century AD), breeders sought balance among the four climate humours. None were to predominate. Breeders believed that Britain's cold, damp climate could be counterbalanced by crossing the Arabian, from a hot and dry climate, on English mares. Mating a horse from the English climate to another horse from that same climate would naturally result in deterioration over generations because of an overbalance of the cold and moist humour. The crossing of an Arabian horse from hot and dry lands could mitigate that effect because the breed was a climate humour opposite to English horses.

The object was not so much to make the English horse lean towards the hot and dry climate type but rather to counteract, or "cancel," the deteriorating effects that doubling up cold on cold would produce. Maintenance and consistency were always at least part of the fundamental objectives. The focus on warding off decline could, however, come to present an ambiguous relationship between maintenance and improvement, as well as between hybridity and purity. William Cavendish (later the Duke of Newcastle) and Lord Fairfax both followed the standard geohumour breeding strategies, but they differed to some degree in what their aims for doing so implied. Cavendish stayed concerned with counteracting the environment to preserve the past. Fairfax hoped to use the ancient method for maintenance but also to manipulate the humours in order to enhance improvement as well.[1] Their attitudes make it clear that it can be difficult to establish neatly what type of motivation divided environmental from improvement breeding. Either maintenance or both maintenance and improvement could be a motivating factor behind a breeder's decision to follow this environmental selection strategy.

Environmental breeding concepts could sometimes lie behind or be hidden in improvement breeding aims after the idea of improvement had become firmly established. The demise of environmental breeding in Western societies did not sound the death knell of beliefs generated by the older system. An example of the continuing impact of environmental breeding and of its interconnection with the motivation to improve can be seen in the views of Federico Tesio, a renowned Italian Thoroughbred horse breeder of the mid-twentieth century. Tesio showed a strong allegiance to seventeenth-century principles of environmental breeding with its often dichotomous objectives, at the same time that he actively tried to improve his racing horses. While he did not overtly support the climate and humour approach, many of his theories echoed other fundamental beliefs held by breeders of earlier times. In 1947 he wrote a book, later translated as *Tesio: In His Own Words*, about his breeding ideology. His curious blend of history, philosophy, Mendelian genetics, and the open desire for improvement along with a seventeenth-century outlook provides a splendid example of how enduring pre-eighteenth-century attitudes could be by the mid-twentieth century. Tesio, for example, spoke of nervous energy in horses, almost as an electric shock from the heavens, and the transmission of that energy via the sexual act. Purity, namely virginity in mares, had an energy of its own, which would be released with sexual meeting with a stallion. That energy, almost a power from the stars, would be transmitted to the foal. Energy he saw as the level of will power in a horse to race with speed. A horse could be too nervous from such energy, however, and in such cases that trend should be counterbalanced through breeding strategies. His sense of balance in breeding closely matched the desire for an avoidance of extremes commonly found in environmental breeding of the seventeenth century. Tesio discussed inbreeding and outcrossing strategies within equine family lines. He also claimed to be devoted to the science of genetics (and he discussed Mendelism in terms of coat colour), but it is entirely evident from his general approach that genetics was not central to his breeding theories.

Tesio presented a basic dichotomy in his conflicting ideas about how the Thoroughbred developed and where its quality came from. His discussion around these issues, while somewhat difficult to follow, reveals something of his allegiance to basic environmental breeding ideology. Effectively, Tesio downplayed the importance of the Arabian for the development of the Thoroughbred and the role that hybrid vigour might have brought, because purity – almost a heavenly gift – was important to him. While he admitted that the Arabian had been part of the makeup of the Thoroughbred (thereby in fact supporting the idea that the breed was a crossbred, or hybrid), Tesio argued that over time all Arabian blood had been completely winnowed out. That implied that the Thoroughbred was pure, and for Tesio purity was a type of perfection which he defined as "resistance" to alteration. Purity meant energy, and a certain inner strength.[2] Rather ambiguously, though, Tesio went on to say that the horses showed improvement in certain desired qualities over the introduced Arabian. Tesio never stated that he adhered to environmental breeding over improvement breeding, but his evident interest in environmentally driven theories suggests a strong fundamental allegiance to the older system. In keeping with Thoroughbred horse culture, however, he also emphasized extreme ancestry breeding.

Evidently an underlying dual approach to maintenance and improvement, as well as to purity and hybridity, could exist in environmental breeding as early as the 1600s and could even persist into the modern period. In certain ways and under varying conditions, the one seemed to partially morph into the other. The two supposedly divergent approaches sometimes bore more in common with each other than meets the eye. That situation provided the seeds for conflict in the twentieth century. The questions became: Which was more important, maintenance or improvement? Did breeding for improvement bring with it deviation from type, which in fact brought about devaluation? In other words, when "improvement" seemed to result in a concurrent decline of a breed's authenticity to historic type, was that in fact degeneration? The wish to preserve "authentic" quality could be seen as more important than the wish to improve that quality. A conflict arose over these questions and pitted one form of breeding ideology against the other. It is important to recognize these realities, because selection with a specialization focus on authenticity became a contentious issue in the breeding of a number of domestic animals. The situations in the Collie (Lassie type) dog and Arabian horse breeding worlds illustrate that general phenomenon. These reviews show that it became more, not less, difficult to distinguish what improvement means in light of the wish to maintain past glories.

Authenticity and Collie (Lassie Type) Breeding

By 1910, English breeders had so changed the phenotype of the old Scottish working sheep dog or "colley," by now known as the Collie, that some Americans began to question the authenticity of the popular modern version. Undesirable qualities in top show dogs fed into the situation. Problems such as narrow heads, perceived to indicate stupidity, temperament problems introduced through inbreeding, and belief in breed impurity owing to the infiltration of Gordon setter or Borzoi genetics were not uncommon by this time.[3] A yearning for the older Collie type made some American buyers look for the type of quality that had been found in early show dogs, believing these dogs represented the original version that existed before contamination. Others thought it would be best to look for non-purebred farm Collies to find what they wanted. A movement to re-establish what was called the old-fashioned Collie arose by 1911 as a result, formally triggered by two letters to the editor of *Country Life in America*. "As long as I can remember," Otis Barnum wrote, "I have heard stories of the wonderful sagacity and faithfulness of Scotch collies, but somehow, since the advent of the modern, sharp-nosed, show type of collies, these stories have been getting fewer … I wish your magazine could do something to save this dog from extinction."[4] A Collie breeder responded to Barnum as follows: "While it is true the present-day collie is different from the old-fashioned type, that does not necessarily imply that he is a degenerate and inferior in every way … The majority of people in this country … have no use for a working dog. They want a dog that is handsome as well as intelligent, and there can be no question of the collie's superlative claims to beauty. He is undoubtedly one of the handsomest, as well as most aristocratic of all our dogs."[5] Fundamentally, the breeder argued that the new version had simply replaced the old one: it was a matter of progress and improvement.

The editor of *Country Life* found the problem posed by these two writers interesting and decided to take up the cause of the old-fashioned Collie. "There is nothing to be gained by discussing the question of superiority between the old and new, because they have become totally different," he wrote in 1912. While the new show Collie was here to stay, the old-fashioned Collie needed to be recognized, perhaps even as a separate breed or type. The newer version should not supplant and replace the older one; what actually had happened was that now two distinct "collie" breeds existed. "We therefore respectfully bring this suggestion to the attention of the authorities of the American Kennel Club, the Collie Club, the Westminster Kennel Club, and any others whose influence is needed to save the old-fashioned collie."[6] Responses from supporters of the new version came in quickly, arguing that it had in fact supplanted the older one. The secretary of the American Kennel Club replied, "I do not understand what you mean by the old-fashioned collie, as there is no such breed." The editor of *International Dogs* said, "Personally I cannot identify the dog you refer to." The important British Collie breeder W.E. Mason wrote to *Country Life* as follows: "I am not clear as to what you mean by the Old-fashioned Collie. If it is that you wish to cultivate the sort that was shown twenty or even less years ago, with thick, coarse heads, light eyes, pendulous ears, and vacant expression, then I am quite sure you will never make any headway and I shall do all I can to show the absurdity of your scheme." The editor of *Country Life* claimed that comments like these simply missed the point. The old-fashioned Collie existed as a separate type or perhaps breed by this stage, and continued to be beloved by many who also stoutly believed in that type's superiority because of its greater authenticity.[7]

Mason decided to pursue the issue in more depth in his *Collie Folio*. "From time to time one hears the wailings and croakings of that portion of the public which believes that the modern Collie is all wrong, and that great retrogression has been the outcome of the labors of those who have striven to improve the grandest of all the canine species. We are amongst those who very much think otherwise." Mason noted that while many might bewail the rise of the new type at the expense of the old, he believed it was irresponsible for the editor of *Country Life* to do so. "Every once in a while someone pops up with a wail and a plea for 'the old-fashioned Collie'. Usually such men are they who have owned stock of the type prevalent in the [18]70's and have done nothing since to improve the points of the breed," Mason stated. But for a reputable journal to take on the cause and promote authenticity against advancements made by breeding was shocking, he added, noting that pictures accompanying *Country Life*'s description of the old-fashioned Collie made "those with an eye for the beautiful ... shudder." Furthermore, Mason argued, the dogs pictured looked very much like Saint Bernards or Newfoundlands, indicating that they might be less pure than the show Collie. The bottom line, Mason said, was that a modern fancy Collie could do anything an old-fashioned Collie could. As far as Mason was concerned, the modern Collie was just the new and improved version of the old.[8]

Many Collie lovers remained unconvinced and sought out the descendants of valuable Collies tracing back to the Victorian era of the 1890s, dogs that ironically were often accused of causing the problem in the first place. Curiously, in light of the attacks made on the financier J.P. Morgan about his role in the breeding of thin-nosed, stupid, non-utility Collies through his demand for high-priced Collie styles, after his death various people wrote to his son, hoping to find in the descendants of Morgan's dogs an old-fashioned utility collie. In 1918, for example, Robert Preston wanted a puppy to replace his beloved pet, descended from a valuable Morgan dog with the "blunter nose which is characteristic of what is called the 'Old Fashioned Collie', now nearly extinct. These dogs ... lacked the treacherous and uncertain temper of the modern sharp nose Collie in addition to being more intelligent."[9] (J.P. Morgan Jr responded that no records of the Collies existed any longer and that the Morgan family did not know what had become of the dogs.)[10] The movement supporting the older version had died down by the 1920s, after editors of journals like *Country Life* and the *Collie Folio* had dropped the subject and probably also partially because the American Kennel Club refused to see the type as a breed. The drive to improve for beauty, and therefore for change, seemed to prevail in most Collie-breeding circles. The movement for authenticity and for preservation of what was perceived to be the original type, however, never entirely disappeared.

Old-fashioned Collies continued to be seen and valued on farms in North America until the late 1950s. By the 1980s, while it had become increasingly difficult to find dogs of this style, admiration for the old-fashioned type had not disappeared. Lovers of the "old fashioned farm Collie," sometimes called the old farm Collie, began a search for those that remained. In 1995, people who had loved these dogs in their childhood, from both the United States and Canada, formed a group called Friends of the Old Farm Collie. They set out to preserve the style's authenticity by re-establishing the old type of collie as a distinct breed. The old-fashioned Collie had recognizable head features – large eyes, ears not too pricked and off the head, and a heavier and wider skull with an evident and pronounced "stop" (where the head domes on dogs like setters). The dog also had shorter legs and a shorter coat. In contrast, the show Collie has smaller eyes, a narrow, tapered head with almost no "stop," and ears with a higher prick and set well up on the head. The legs are longer, as is the body, and the coat is much longer. Fans of the old collie type began publishing a bulletin on the Internet that recorded their progress.[11]

Some members of Friends of the Old Farm Collie decided that their ideal for an old-fashioned Collie closely resembled the early bench show Collies of the 1880s, and they formed the Classic Victorian Collie Club.[12] By the late 1990s, the move to create the older type of Collie had taken a more formalized shape. The American Working Farmcollie Association had also been established with a registration system, making the old-fashioned Collie a "purebred" breed, even if the American Kennel Club did not accept it as such.[13] How much this "new" breed actually represents authenticity to true type, because of the fluidity in defining what era created true type, remains an open question. The very division of farm collie from Victorian collie serves as an example of how such definitions can splinter. People have continued, regardless of difficulties in definitions as seen in the Victorian collie movement, to support the older versions. The Association's mission statement claims that the organization "is a performance registry dedicated to the preservation and conservation of the traditional working farm dog of Collie ancestry."[14] Pedigree registration proceeds under certain set standards qualifying animals as the Working Farmcollie. Aficionados share images and information on the Internet, and breed varieties of the dogs as well.[15] The continuation of interest in the old farm collie and ongoing resistance to the idea that the modern show Collie alone – vastly changed since the late 1990s in style – represents the true "collie" type serve as an example of much underlying disenchantment many people have with the entire Kennel Club system, its definition of "breed," and its breed specialty clubs which set the written standards.

The old-fashioned Collie movement stimulated discussion for and against the idea of authenticity and consequently maintenance of type in relation to both quality and improvement. Clearly, those supporting authenticity had a vision that was not closely linked with monetary concerns. It is interesting too, though, that the reactions against the movement by those seeking to change the dogs and make them into a better and more modern model of the older type reveal an aesthetic vision behind their breeding aim. Commentary made by these breeders can also be detached from self-serving commercial interests. Both sides presented almost crusade-like features in their thinking.

The Arabian Horse and Authenticity as a Breeding Aim

The history of an authenticity debate in Arabian horse breeding that erupted in the mid-twentieth century shows that notions concerning original type could be much more complicated when attempts to define it rested on the idea that the Eastern and the Western breeding ethos should be viewed together. Eastern breeding heritage, which entailed exotic ideas (from a Western point of view) about both how to keep track of ancestry and how to follow breeding strategies, fascinated Western breeders. Compounding these matters, however, was the fact that the Arabs had functioned under the ethos of environmental breeding, not Western-style improvement breeding. Defining improvement in relation to environmental breeding and contingently authenticity to type would, therefore, be particularly challenging. Since understanding the breeding practices of ancient Arab peoples would be central to any debate around authenticity, it is important to outline what we know about their selection strategies.[16]

The Bedouin breeders kept track of what were called "strains" in the horses. Strains defined the family line an individual horse belonged to, revealing its genealogy in a certain way. One particularly significant characteristic of Arab strain recording was its emphasis on female lines. The Arabs kept track of their breeding families within the strain relation of mares, not stallions. It is not clear, though, whether the ancient Bedouins practised strain breeding, or whether strain breeding involved either inbreeding, or pure in strain breeding. It is not clear either how or why the concept of strains developed in the first place. Importantly, strain theory did fit with the idea of purity, which came to mean trueness to correct type and the preservation of that type through restriction of incoming equine blood. Arab breeding techniques might have charmed Turks, Egyptians, western Europeans, and Americans for centuries, but records left by such travellers to Arabia or other Islamic countries (particularly those collected in the nineteenth century) provided unclear accounts about the nature of Bedouin practices or how attitudes to strain fitted with those practices.[17]

Perhaps even more important, there seemed also to be little contemporary appreciation by Western writers of the fact that by the nineteenth century Bedouin and Western views about selection were divided by Arab adherence to environmental breeding versus Western adherence to improvement breeding. The hidden and shifting environmental-to-improvement factor would, it turned out much later, take on considerable significance. When an authenticity focus became prevalent in mid-twentieth-century Arabian horse breeding in the United States and Europe, misunderstandings about the nature of historical transitions in Western historical thinking about breeding became critical. Comprehending how purity fitted into strain theory and how strain theory fitted with recording or breeding methodology would be difficult, and often contentious as well, among different groups of Western breeders.

Considerable evidence can be discerned in contemporary writings – even if the underlying implications were not dwelt on by diarists – to support the contention that the Bedouin breeders sought to preserve or reinforce desired type rather than seek improvement. The nineteenth-century writings of Western travellers in particular corroborate the contention that preservation of type dominated Bedouin breeding.[18] Young foals, Westerners found, were deprived of water for their first few days of life for unclear reasons, but possibly the custom arose to test foal stamina in the environment. (Arabia is a hot dry country.) Seasons dictated when to breed and which animal should be bred more than any outward appreciation of quality in an individual. Bedouins believed in telegony – namely that if a mare carried a foal by an undesirable stallion (usually simply meaning one owned by a foreign tribe), all her future foals sired by different stallions would be tainted. It is not difficult to see how telegony concepts would shape views about her strain (or sub-strain). Because only mares that had never been covered by the wrong horse were of the highest quality, the strain of such mares would easily become connected with quality. By inference, if a mare was clean she was also pure. Foals born from the wrong crossing became, like their dams, valueless for breeding purpose and therefore were also of low quality.[19]

For Western breeders of the mid-twentieth century, attempts to understand Bedouin breeding focused primarily on appreciating the methodology used at the Arabian studs of nineteenth-century Egypt, particularly those of Abbas Pasha and the last significant stud owned by the breeder Ali Pasha Sherif. The main reason that horses from this latter stud, and their breeding, were so important to Western people was the fact that it had been built on the earlier one of Abbas Pasha, who collected horses from the desert and housed one thousand animals at his stud's height.[20] Anything that had been written by Abbas Pasha or Ali Pasha Sherif, as well as any information attributed to them, became highly significant, and in many ways even surpassed what had been learned directly from Bedouin breeders in Arabia.[21] Of supreme importance to the drive for authenticity, though, would be how faithful either Egyptian breeder had been to breeding strategies practised in the desert. Discussion that took place in the twentieth century over what authenticity breeding meant often hinged on that one point. The important and fundamental questions for many Western breeders would be: What was Abbas Pasha's goal in breeding? Did he want to maintain the true authenticity of the horse of the desert? Abbas Pasha might receive credit for preserving the authenticity of the Arabian, but there is evidence that his breeding practices reflected his personal vision of what authenticity meant or should be.

It has been argued that Abbas Pasha altered the original Bedouin horse even while he claimed he was trying to protect both purity and authenticity, by selecting desert horses on the basis of his perception of beauty, the dished face being particularly significant. Later authors believed that Bedouin breeders did not see the dished face as desirable and that in the future it came to dominate all Arabian horse breeding because of Abbas Pasha's obsession with it. As one authenticity breeder stated much later, "breaking the Occidental breeder – or buyer – of the conviction that the Arabian horse and a dished face are synonymous" is virtually impossible; she added, "it is not an attribute of the purebred Arabian but a throwback to the Abbas Pasha early selections from the desert."[22] Abbas Pasha also tended to favour horses for their ability to sprint, and he bred for that characteristic too. Animals admired by the Bedouins reflected a concern for preserving the animals' innate endurance qualities rather than increasing their capacity for short speed. Furthermore, Bedouin breeders wanted to safeguard the natural tendency of the horses to go far on little food and water.[23] Abbas bred, it appears, for what he believed to be improvement of original type. He did not, however, completely abandon the conviction that the environment played a role in maintaining both the quality of individuals and their ability to breed to that quality, even if he selected for a type personally admired by him. Note what he said in 1852 to Baron Von Huegal, a buyer for the famous Weil Stud (established in 1817) in Germany: "Never for a moment must you believe that the horses born in your countries are genuine Arabs, for the simple reason that the Arab horse can scarcely retain its quality and characteristics for which it is renowned unless it breathes the desert air."[24] Clearly Abbas Pasha believed that the environment played a role in stamping authenticity as to the phenotype. While he was not alone in believing that animals degenerated over generations when taken from their place of origin, something more than that conviction seems to underlie his words.[25]

Abbas Pasha's vision related to preserving authenticity through breeding done on Eastern terms and in the East in order to maintain quality already built in.

In 1854 Abbas Pasha was assassinated, and with the dispersal of the famous stud in 1860 Ali Pasha Sherif became the owner of its greatest and most influential part.[26] Ali Pasha Sherif's stud would be the last reservoir of Abbas Pasha genetics, and therefore the breeding techniques of Abbas Pasha became incorporated into those of Ali Pasha Sherif. When Ali Pasha Sherif's sons dispersed the remnants of the breeding centre in 1897, the genetics of these horses entered European breeding centres in greater numbers than they had in earlier times.[27] Wilfrid and Anne Blunt, owners of the Crabbet Arabian stud in England, had this to say about the stud and its horses in those final days. "We saw Ali Pasha's Stud in the last years of its disruption. Decimated by plague and weakened by years of inbreeding and gross neglect, the horses were of an ethereal quality and truly like gazelles, with no more bone. It was 'Type' etherealized almost to extinction."[28] The Blunts built their new Arabian stud partially on lines from the last of Ali Pasha Sherif stock and partially on animals that they had bought from Bedouins in the desert. While they kept their horses pure to Eastern ancestry, they did not devote themselves to strain breeding.

In the early part of the twentieth century, the operation passed to the hands of Wilfrid and Anne Blunt's daughter, Judith Blunt Lytton (later Lady Wentworth), who took centre stage in the Western world of Arabian horse breeding. She openly resisted attempting to follow the potential breeding theories of Abbas Pasha and subsequently Ali Pasha Sherif. Like her parents before her, Wentworth did not breed by strain, and she believed that the Bedouins had not done so either. She wanted to alter original type, even if within pure lines, because she considered improvement more important than maintaining authenticity to what she believed was faulty type. When some accused her of diverging from authentic style, Wentworth responded: "If being 'off-type' means having higher withers, longer rein and curve of neck, stronger and broader quarters and better hocks, together with freer hock action, then I am proud to say that I have deliberately bred for these points and shall continue to do so."[29] Good foundation animals could and should be bred to produce better stock. Wentworth's breeding philosophy laid the groundwork for the dominant approaches to breeding and to the meaning of authenticity that prevailed until mid-century. In effect she established what might be called the Wentworth authenticity version of Arabian horse breeding, which was based to some degree on the research carried out by her mother, Lady Anne Blunt.[30] The Wentworth views would be challenged in the 1950s by what could be defined as the Raswan authenticity approach.

American breeders interested in the new form of authenticity relied heavily on Carl Raswan's work on Bedouin breeding – his book and his horse index. Born in Germany in 1893, Raswan (whose name had been Carl Reinhardt Schmidt) travelled extensively in Arabia during the years around the First World War. He became an American citizen in 1927, changing his name to that of a favourite Arabian stallion (ironically, not from pure Bedouin stock) bred by Lady Wentworth. He wrote about breeding techniques of the Arab people while living in the United States, long after his travels in Arabia. He put forward the theory that there were only three overarching strains (all with numerous sub-strains), which represented three distinct physical types within the single breed. The three strain types were the Saklawi (refined, elegant, and feminine), the Kuhaylan (powerful, bold, and masculine), and the Muniqi (with a racier build and usually with the forequarters more developed than the hindquarters).[31] (These names have a variety of English spellings.)

Raswan believed that the Arabs had practised strain breeding and also inbreeding. He argued that in order for modern Arabians to maintain their trueness to authentic type, they should be bred within strain, using inbreeding to stay in strain. Raswan also held certain convictions about the value of the three strains. All breeding should be away from the Muniqi strain, which he claimed was impure as a result of one Bedouin cross with a Turkish stallion in the seventeenth century. A pure or *asil* Arabian had no Muniqi blood. Raswan stated that Europeans had in the past favoured Muniqis because of their racing ability, and that had stimulated their production for the European market. (The Darley Arabian, probably the most important founder of the Thoroughbred, had been a Muniqi.) Raswan believed that, for their own purposes, the Bedouins did not breed to Muniqi if they could help it.[32]

The Raswan version of authenticity made some breeders particularly obsessed with descendants of Ali Pasha Sherif stock because of their background in Abbas Pasha breeding, or with other animals descended from stock bought in the desert. Major establishments devoted to breeding by strain in order to maintain purity to Bedouin breeding, or to Abbas Pasha based breeding through that stock, came into existence. As one traditional American breeder noted in 1958 in reaction to the authenticity trend: "Dazzled by the fiery elegance, the stylish bearing and the fabled history of the Arabian horse, some fanciers of the breed have naively insisted that the Arab is and always has been 'perfect' and that any attempt to improve on that perfection would be presumptuous."[33] The three strains defined as Saklawi, Kuhaylan, and Muniqi took on new meaning under these conditions. The passion for purity and authenticity to Arab standards, combined with extensive American and European importing from countries that held ancient Arabian breeding centres, had in effect reawakened the whole issue of strains and authenticity and triggered a reaction against the dominant breeding trend in Arabians that had been initiated by the Blunts and further established by Lady Wentworth.

The renewed interest in strains that resulted from Raswan's work made some American breeders start to categorize modern Arabians in relation particularly to their origins from Arabia, Blunt, or Abbas Pasha stock (found in Ali Pasha Sherif breeding). "Blue star" described horses that descended on all sides from these roots and with no Muniqi blood. "Blue list" animals traced to these roots as well, but with 1 to 50 per cent breeding of Muniqi. All other Arabians were "general list."[34] These new studs, which were well established by the 1950s, practised inbreeding within strain and away from Muniqi to preserve true type. Breeders claimed that perpetuating type defined the highest quality and that any attempts at improvement – beauty for one thing – meant degradation. "The challenge of authenticity breeding has not been in the production of good horses because this has resulted from the automatic biological process," one breeder specializing in pure Bedouin background stock explained. As far as this breeder was concerned, the challenge was convincing people that the truly authentic Arabian was the most superior type.[35] Raswan authenticity breeders argued that most American Arabian horse breeding since the early part of the century – and particularly as a result of favouring the animals of Lady Wentworth and her breeding approaches – had ended up with a mass of non-authentic Arabians. As Kathleen Ott wrote: "The poly glot animals that ... sprung up to supply the demand for a pretty show horse and something that approximated the highly stylized paintings of the old romantics ... [have] resulted in a diversion from the original Arabian, with a corresponding loss of Arab quality."[36]

There was a strong reaction from those who had devoted years and knowledge to the breeding of Arabians on the basis of the Wentworth authenticity version and who believed in striving for superior type – particularly better-structured legs – while maintaining the head and neck characteristics so desirable in Arabians. Beauty, style, usefulness, and structural soundness were important to them, and in their defence of their breeding aims, they reveal a side of the breeding industry that clearly adhered to more than the pursuit of markets. The dream of improvement over environmental breeding seemed to underlie much of their motivation to breed. Note the statement of one improvement breeder in California. "Study of strains within the Arabian breed, their origins and their alleged characteristics, is intriguing, often fascinating, and occasionally amusing, but in this modern day, application of the Bedouin system of horse breeding would only be stepping backward into another world and another century."[37] Gladys Brown Edwards, a renowned scholar on the history and breeding of Arabians who worked for the W.K. Kellogg Arabian breeding centre in California over the 1930s and early 1940s, became a major spokesperson for the Wentworth version, or what might be called its American counterpart, the combined Wentworth Kellogg version.

Edwards was outraged by this turn of events, which supported the disfavour of improvement breeding, and particularly objected to Raswan's theory concerning the Muniqi strain. "The [Muniqi] is no more 'angular' than is any other strain," she wrote, "mainly because there is no such thing as a 'strain type' other than [that] now assigned it by 'authorities' who find it easy to do so by 'looks' and not by actual strain and this mainly because of the 'Raswan Theory' now completely discredited ... At any rate, the [Muniqi] was no more 'impure' than any other, and Raswan's vague story about one obscure tribe crossing with 'Turcoman stallions' (he first said one, then kept adding to them – himself – not the tribe – though on paper of course[)] – and pow! – automatically all [Muniqi] horses in Arabia became contaminated! Even he finally could not swallow that and in later years took part of it back."[38] Edwards passionately led the crusade against the Raswan anti-improvement and authenticity movement by writing articles in Arabian horse magazines. "To Progress ... or Regress That Is the Question," she wrote in the *Arab Horse Journal*, and asked fellow breeders, "is your horse descended from certain celebrated individuals or has it ascended from them?" She continued, deriding the "Anties," as she called the new style of authenticity-driven breeders, because they seemed so "anti" any Arabian not derived from and duplicating, as they defined it, pure Bedouin breeding:

> To look down on [show winners who arise from the ranks of the improved Arabian] because they do not trace in every line to either Abbas Pasha blood or to horses direct from the desert and with therefore untraceable pedigrees, is not only unfair to good horses, but is also unrealistic and foolish ... Although we are told by the Cult of the [Anties] to forget utility, beauty, and conformation and breed only for "blood" (of their idea of authenticity), I rather doubt if this will be regarded seriously enough by the majority of breeders to cause a degeneration – i.e.

> "descent" in the quality of European and American Arabians by following such a course ... The horses of Abbas Pasha breeding have generally been accepted as being of high quality, having been bred from known pedigree for several generations, towards a fixed type ... The fact that many of the Abbas Pasha stock were of known (and written) pedigree is the only reason the "classic strain" people have for their claim that these animals are now the only Arabians of absolutely pure blood and no "violent" [Muniqi] crosses. However many of these pedigrees stop abruptly in the Desert.

And furthermore, she stated, "to scrap such benefit and regress into yesteryear does not seem in accord with American initiative and progress."[39] Improvement breeding and the systems designed to bring about improvement had clearly, as far as she was concerned, replaced the more antiquated and backward thinking and methods that had dominated Europe up until the eighteenth century.

Edwards's views were shaped by the background of the Kellogg ranch, which had been given to the state of California in 1932. She inherited a rich culture of Arabian horse breeding which reflected the combined Wentworth and Kellogg authenticity version – one which also provides a clear example of breeding being devoted to love (or passion) for the animals and not to monetary gain. Her attitudes to Raswan were coloured by what had happened when the ranch's founder, W.K. Kellogg (of cereal fame), established his breeding establishment in 1925. At that time Kellogg, by his own admission, knew little about horses and next to nothing about how to breed. These facts brought him into the world of Raswan, who became his purchasing agent, and through Raswan to Wentworth's breeding at Crabbet. Kellogg had an unusual dream when he began his Arabian horse operation, even though he had no knowledge about actual breeding. He wanted not only to preserve the authenticity of the Arabian via purity but also to combine that purity with professional efforts at improving the best of the original type. Furthermore, Kellogg wanted to pursue his breeding venture, not for his benefit, but rather for the benefit of the United States. From the beginning, he had planned to eventually hand it over as a gift to the state of California supplied by endowment funds. Making money was clearly not his objective. As he wrote in an unsent letter to Lady Wentworth: "I did not engage in this business for the purpose of pure profit, but in the hope that I might be of some service to the World in propagating these wonderful animals, and in doing so I hoped to derive considerable pleasure."[40] Kellogg elaborated on his plans and his reliance on Raswan in the following letter, which he did send to Wentworth in April 1926, early in their relationship.

> I believe it will be possible to so frame up [a] Trust Deed, that the Arab horses will be thereby protected, and instructions concerning their breeding etc., carried out specifically … I hope to live many years to enjoy these wonderful animals; but while I feel that I am too old to be initiated into all degrees of the mysteries pertaining to the Arab horses, trust that I may live a sufficient length of time to see this wonderful breed established in America … I am depending on Carl Schmidt [later Raswan] to pass along his enthusiasm to … scientific horse breeders … and am in hopes that all of our plans and desires be completely carried out … I am depending upon Schmidt to assist me … I shall be glad at all future times to co-operate with you in the plans you have for saving the Arab horses.[41]

Both Kellogg and Wentworth quickly came to see that Raswan, while he appeared to know something about Arabians and certainly was almost obsessed with them, seemed to have unclear reasons for being involved with the horses. Raswan might have set himself up as a partner with the two in the mission to save the pure Arabian, but the lack of clarity and the complexity of his motives made it difficult to see how that could be the case. He seemed removed from the preservation and at the same time improvement vision of Kellogg, as well as holding different views concerning purity and authenticity from those of Wentworth. Furthermore, his business relations with the two were muddied by clearly unethical behaviour. By June of 1926, for example, Kellogg had become aware that Raswan had used Kellogg funds without permission.[42] Kellogg subsequently fired Raswan, reporting to Wentworth as follows: "I wish to state to you quite definitely that I do not want you to do anything whatsoever for me thru Carl Schmidt [Raswan]; my business relations that we may enter into will be direct; my experiences with Schmidt have been most unhappy and vexatious."[43]

Wentworth had had her private concerns about Raswan from the beginning. To begin with, she did not naturally trust agents, stating to Kellogg that August that she "hate[d] and deteste[d] paid agents." "They are always crooks," she added. Raswan, she now believed, had always misled her. "I am more and more astonished and horrified at the way in which I have been misled by C. Schmidt. I find that the opinions which made me think he knew about horses were prompted by someone else and he came here already primed," she confided to her son, Captain Milbanke.[44] As far as Wentworth was concerned, both

Kellogg's and her own reputation were at stake as a result of Raswan's behaviour. "I am distressed at S's mad attempt to wreck your enterprise and my reputation as a breeder," she stated; "I am surprised that you retain the smallest interest in the Arab horse. Few people would do so after such an experience."[45]

Evidently the experiences of Kellogg and Wentworth with Raswan in the 1920s diverged significantly from views concerning his passion for Arabians held by proponents of the Raswan authenticity vision in the 1950s. The man apparently had a complex character. It is worth noting, though, that, while many Americans might have become enamoured with Raswan's vision by the 1950s, Kellogg and Wentworth were not the only breeders in the 1920s who distrusted the man after direct contacts with him through the employer relationship. One such person was the renowned American breeder W.R. Brown, who had been concerned with improving the stamina of horses for the armed forces from at least 1910 and believed that the pure Arabian could infuse that quality into homebred American horses of different backgrounds.[46] An importer of Crabbet stock from the time of the Blunts, Brown hired Raswan in 1929 to accompany him to the desert in search of true Arabian horses. Their association did not last long, as Brown explained to Kellogg in June of that year. "You would be interested to hear that I have just fired Raswan. I left him with $2,500 in Beirut, the first money I trusted him with, to ship my horses home and he spent it for manuscripts in Cairo, and misappropriated it in many ways ... He skipped out and I located him at Lady Wentworth's, presumably to find a sale for the manuscripts which he had bought with my money, or sell her some information."[47] For unknown reasons, the animals Brown bought with Raswan as agent in Arabia never reached the United States.

The authenticity conflict of the late 1950s and 1960s offers an interesting look at how Western improvement breeders viewed not only the nature of authenticity but also (and at a deeper level) the older and largely supplanted environmental breeding, which had declined – at least in the Western world – with changes in naturalist attitudes to the process of heredity. Although breeders rarely if ever articulated the issue in that fashion, it is hard to escape the suspicion that in essence the authenticity versus improvement debate rested on certain unanswered, albeit hidden, questions. Did improvement breeding define breeding for quality? Did environmental breeding not reflect breeding for quality? Was quality even an aspect of a breeding methodology? How did authenticity or uniformity fit into this picture? The tensions between the authenticity and improvement breeders over such difficulties might be explained by, first, a basic misunderstanding by all of them of what underlying theories drove both environmental and improvement breeding, and, second (more importantly), a lack of appreciation for the way the two systems related to and contrasted with each other. It was misleading, for example, to differentiate the two on the basis of selection being used as a breeding strategy. Improvement breeding cannot be defined by its adherence to selective breeding, as was (and is) commonly done.[48] Selection has always been as much a part of environmental as improvement systems. Bedouin breeding might have been an effort at maintenance but, like all environmental methods, it also reflected selective breeding. Similarities of this nature seemed to escape the comprehension of Arabian horse breeders in Western countries.

Breeders who focused on authenticity seemed to take an almost crusade-like approach to breeding, as opposed to the commercial outlook common to improvement breeding. Authenticity breeders might be driven by a yearning for the past or a sense of the exotic, but their motivation to breed was not that different from that of improvement breeders. While clashes took place with breeders who sought change and improvement (and who took an attitude to breeding more in line with Enlightenment thinking), the improvement breeders were driven, at least to some extent, by similar crusade-like aims and non-market forces. Kellogg himself presents the strongest example of non-commercial motivation for breeding.

The fire driving authenticity breeding seemed to die down or take a new turn by the late 1970s. The American Arabian horse world developed internal fractures which supported styles developed in Egypt, Russia, Poland, and Sweden, and also older American lines, along with Crabbet and Wendworth breeding. Interest in foreign genetics in the United States only increased the desire of American breeders to buy abroad. Investors too were attracted by these lines. Tax reforms in 1986 led to a collapse of the hot Arabian horse market worldwide, which had been driven by American demand. When the dust had settled, the move back to authenticity and reverence for historic strain theory gathered new momentum. By the 1990s the authenticity drive became focused again on Egyptian Arabians, especially those descended from Abbas Pasha stock. Authenticity people had predicted in the 1950s that such a thing would happen. The belief that Abbas Pasha stock and subsequently Ali Pasha Sherif stock was 100 per cent Bedouin breeding and 100 per cent pure (no Muniqi blood) made breeders as early as the 1960s turn to older, pure Egyptian lines in order to get back to what they believed was true type. "Their preference for the Egyptian type [had become] so pronounced that 'Egyptian breeding' threatened to become a cult," one person wrote (prophetically) at that time, adding the following: "With breeders depending on '50% Egyptian breeding' or less to undo every mistake European and American breeders have ever made."[49]

Authenticity, not improvement, was, in effect, the gold standard for supporters of Egyptian stock. When one of the most prominent advocates of Egyptian horses, and also one of the earliest American importers in the 1950s, was asked if the breed even could be improved, the answer was an emphatic and clearly worded environmental and at the same time authenticity statement. "No," she said. "The standard was established thousands of years ago."[50] How selection strategies fit into authenticity and maintenance breeding seems to warrant little written attention from the modern breeders of Egyptian Arabians. At least, they do not emphasize such things, perhaps partially because they do not want to reopen the conflicts that related most directly to Raswan and his Muniqi/Turkoman theories. Authenticity could be had outside Raswan's convictions about the value of particular strains. The new authenticity focus on Egyptian Arabians rapidly expanded over the late 1990s to become global in nature. (The market implications of breeding for authenticity will be dealt with in chapter 8.)

The review of breeding aims reveals interesting ways people related to animals, how that relationship has changed, and what factors play a role in shifts. These issues are separate from how to develop methodology or how science might impact practical breeding. Methodology would be used to achieve improvement through selection for various characteristics, but methodology did not define what improvement meant or dictate what should be improved. How to breed became blurred with reasons to breed, so it is often difficult to see what the major drivers behind either actually were. One factor driving selection strategies was levels of technology. In the case of North American dairying, factory cheese making and creamery butter became the critical factors in initiating the ultimate drive for specialized dairy cattle breeding, the separation of beef from dairy emphasis. In the Netherlands, the same factory structure also drove increased specialization for milk yields in cattle already bred to that purpose. Horse breeding for traction purposes tended to be driven by technological developments that splintered haulage needs. Shifting traction needs resulted from the enormous changes brought about by industrialization and the growth of cities. Farmers found it hard to breed for various horse types, however, because it was difficult to keep up with the increasingly divided demands made by industrial developments. A move to breeding for increased size and weight in all horses, for use on the farm or off, evolved from that situation. Ultimately technology in the form of the internal combustion engine brought about the demise of the working horse altogether.

Beauty or fancy specialization might appear to be a driver of selection for colour, but this trend, like others, could relate to markets as well as to culture and knowledge of genetics, and a review of nineteenth- to twenty-first-century Collie breeding reveals this intertwined complexity. Basic views regarding what was beautiful remained unchanged, in spite of better knowledge of genetics and in spite of an appreciation for colour derivatives from the genetic base causing all-white. Colour could also relate to the way industry structure worked, made evident in the Colour Craze in late nineteenth-century Shorthorns. Marketability of uniform colour drove the interest in red Shorthorns, through the chain from feeders to cow/calf operators to bull suppliers in the American Midwest, and had a reverberating effect on breeders in Canada. Breeding for colour could be connected with the act of breeding as a sport. The complicated system designed to produce perfection of colour in the American Barred Plymouth Rock was as much about the skill in breeding as it was about colour itself. Breeding for colour dictated what breed of poultry would dominate hybrid breeding for egg production, because different breeds produced eggs of different colours. Consumer preference became the driver.

Real passion for animals runs through breeding for authenticity. And respect as well. Breeding to avoid manipulation, believed to be contaminated by ideas of commercialism (rampant in the dog fancy),[51] became almost an ethical issue. These concepts also reflected the sense that efforts at improvement meant degeneration of historic type. The dream of authenticity, unlike that relating to economic purpose, did not arise from a gendered position: both men and women could support it. The philosophic and ethical bent of authenticity breeding also lends itself to the idea that not all breeding solely reflected monetary interests. The only monetary gain for many authenticity breeders would be from within the pool of fellow believers. (Of course, the more widespread that pool might be, the greater the financial implications would be, as will be seen in chapter 8.) A desire to recapture the glory of bygone days seemed to characterize aspects of the authenticity vision. The passion for authenticity, however, often aroused the scorn of breeders devoted to improvement as the mantra of general advancement found in modernity and in the predominant improvement breeding of the times, which had replaced environmental breeding in the eighteenth century. There appears to be something aesthetic, however, about both authenticity and improvement views.

Breeding aims could be both complicated and focused on many issues, but another major factor in animal breeding is how it has been regulated and organized over time. The next section shows that the orchestration and regulation of breeding played a significant role in the way we use animals, and circulate them and the ideas that went into their breeding. How, in effect, have we marketed animals? It will be evident from following section that trade regulations have been an important influence on the value of animals, what aims we breed towards, and why we use certain methods to achieve both ends.

SECTION THREE

Orchestrating Breeding: Pedigrees and Trade

Chapter Seven

Pedigree versus No Pedigree and the Market Value of Animals

Purebred breeding orchestrated the affairs of breeding animals through publicly recorded pedigrees, which defined the value of true or pure lines. The longstanding connection of pedigree keeping with the purity versus quality dilemma, however, played a critical role in hiding its most important function. In the end pedigrees' greatest effect was on trade in animals. The regulatory function pedigrees had in defining "breeds," shaping markets, and directing trade would be critical to how livestock markets functioned. It was not always clear, however, how well breeders themselves understood that reality. This section addresses pedigree keeping in relation to all these issues. The idea that pedigrees were a marketing device, it should be pointed out, is not new in academic literature.[1] What is new is the presentation here of a panorama of trade patterns, in considerable detail, which reveal how and why that was the case, but equally important what the ramifications of those trade-driven trends could be. Looking at a number of situations that took place involving cattle and horses with pedigrees makes clear not only that pedigrees and their standards could create "breeds" and skew the market but also that they could do so in various ways. This chapter looks at the trade and pedigree axis by assessing value in animals in relation to their having pedigrees versus their not having pedigrees.

Early Shorthorns and Pedigrees

Value in connection with pedigree and the purebred system became evident first, logically, in the Shorthorn world because these cattle were the original purebred species known as such. When Felix Renick of the Ohio Importing Company decided in 1833 to buy only cattle with pedigrees while on his shopping expedition in England, the market importance of purebred breeding and its system of pedigree keeping was confirmed. Holding a pedigree was the single most important criterion he used in his selection. Good stock without pedigrees he passed by. As he wrote home to the shareholders:

> The value depends almost entirely upon the purity of the blood and high pedigree ... Thus you see the situation we are placed in. We must take either cattle without pedigree or much of anything else to recommend them or take those that have at least pedigrees, with more excellence of form and size, at a higher price. The latter was in our judgment the better of the two alternatives and the one we have so far pursued, and shall continue to pursue, and take fewer in number ... We want none without fair pedigrees, but form and size they must have or they will not be well received here.[2]

This was an innovative decision. Renick was aware that excellent, non-pedigreed Shorthorns were well appreciated at that time in the United States, descendants of 1817 English importations by Kentucky cattlemen. Described as the Seventeens, and known for their quality, the animals did not carry publicly recorded pedigrees because in 1817 there was no public record-keeping system for cattle.[3] Renick recognized that the cattle trade had changed by 1833 and he believed that, to protect the shareholders' investments, he should focus on stock with pedigrees under a public recording system. Certification and documentation of hereditary background had entered the world of practical breeding. Because the Shorthorn was the single breed with a public herd book in 1833, Renick bought Shorthorns. He purchased Bates cattle (a decision with lasting significance for American Shorthorns until the end of the century), including a few Duchesses, animals descended from and inbred to an original cow by that name. Renick's view proved to be the correct one. Apparently buying pedigree did pay. When the Ohio Importing Company auctioned off the stock, that fact became evident to all.

An elaborate catalogue, containing complete pedigrees of the animals offered, accompanied the first sale held in 1836. Some thirty-three head sold at an average of about $800 per animal. The 1837 dispersal sale of the last of the stock, fifteen cattle, realized an even higher average: roughly $1000 a head. These prices were remarkable when compared with yearly incomes in Ohio country at that time; $200 would have been impressive. Proceeds from these sales generated about $50,000, a good profit for the shareholders' $9,200 investment.[4] But the investors made an even better profit than that, because they kept some of the stock they bought (or calves born from those animals). While the reputation of the newly acquired Shorthorns rose, that of the Seventeens fell (and with serious ramifications for some Canadian breeders seventy years later). Ironically, the cattle that had stimulated the formation of the Ohio Importing Company lost their exalted position when the newcomers arrived, simply because the Seventeens did not have recorded pedigrees. The Renick story concerning Shorthorns shows the importance of pedigrees to marketing, a pattern laid down by the public pedigreeing of the Thoroughbred horse. It was a pattern that would continue, regardless of the more elaborate structures that came into existence with respect to regulation of breeding via pedigrees. It did not take long, though, for pedigrees to be graded against each other.

A Market Bubble: The Shorthorn "Duchess" Debacle and Pedigrees

A particularly hot livestock bubble that emerged in the mid-nineteenth century demonstrates how certain pedigrees could be seen to be especially valuable and how that fact could drive the market. Shortly after 1850, wealthy businessmen saw the buying and selling of certain Shorthorn cattle, because of their pedigrees, as investments in a lucrative livestock market. By 1860 what was described as a full-blown pedigree craze (a phenomenon that bore a strong resemblance to the hot tulipomania craze of the seventeenth century in Holland) had developed in trade patterns between wealthy businessmen collecting Shorthorns in Britain and North America. It was initiated by the situation in Britain, where breeders followed an extremely intense inbreeding strategy for Bates's Duchess-line animals.[5] In the United States, Kentucky cattlemen had also developed a strong interest in Bates's Duchess genetics.[6] An ensuing shortage of Duchess cattle in Britain, owing to excessive inbreeding, provided Americans with a lucrative market for animals with specific pedigrees.

Complicated trade patterns quickly led to a bubble. Several individuals at that time became part of the rapidly developing international Duchess Shorthorn situation. Wealthy New York businessmen Samuel Thorne and J.O. Sheldon, for example, found they had a healthy market for their Duchesses in Britain, a fact which might have encouraged Mathew Cochrane, a Canadian senator from the Eastern Townships of Quebec, to invest in Duchess cattle. He began buying them through his manager, Simon Beattie.[7] Cochrane's move into the market at this particular time drove up prices on a scarce commodity just when several wealthy men in New York, particularly Samuel Campbell, started to amass herds of pure Duchesses on the basis of the Thorne but more particularly Sheldon herds.

Campbell's adviser, Richard Gibson, encouraged Campbell to invest in Duchess stock. In 1873 Gibson decided that the speculation in Duchess cattle had reached a peak and he recommended that Campbell sell out. Buyers converged for the sale of the world's largest herd of living Duchesses. One, Eighth Duchess of Geneva, was sold to an Englishman for $40,600, at a time when yearly incomes in North America averaged less than $500. An observer wrote, "One long breath, and then the cheers went up, and thousands there seemed fairly beside themselves, and extravagant things which were said and done would fill a volume."[8] Many agricultural people watched the sale and the earlier evolution of the Duchess craze with shocked fascination. "The vast proportion of those who have read the newspaper reports of the proceedings of sale heartily unite in setting down the purchasers at it, as a body of hopeless lunatics," commented the *Farmer's Advocate* in Canada.[9] Within a few days, the cow delivered a stillborn heifer, and she herself died shortly thereafter. Surprisingly, the market for Duchess cattle did not break with the New York Mills sale and the debacle around the cow's death. In fact it did not collapse until the loans procured to buy the expensive cattle began to come due. Kentucky breeders continued to buy the stock as long as they could. But infertility due to inbreeding finally took the ultimate toll. By 1883, regardless of whether or not a market existed for them, none of the cattle remained. Pure Duchesses had become extinct.[10]

Cattle breeders remembered the sale over the years with horror. In 1897 the president of the Shorthorn association in Canada called the sale "one of the worst days in Shorthorn history."[11] The Duchess craze made it clear to everyone just how much pedigrees mattered, and how they could be misinterpreted. There was no pretending that animals counted more than pedigrees when it was clear that pedigrees in this case were far more important than animals. Pedigrees, apparently, could take on a life of their own above and beyond the animal: they could be graded against each other through the inbreeding and purity linkage, and to a level beyond anything Bates would have dreamt of, let alone Bakewell. The extreme devotion to pedigree and to inbreeding rarely reached that height again (even though both remained important underlying features of purebred breeding methodology until well into the twentieth century), but the importance of pedigrees alone, with no reference to the quality of an animal for value, could continue and even grow after the Duchess debacle. The powerful link between pedigree and market quickly led to the growth of false pedigrees being peddled because of the worth that any pedigrees, regardless of quality, had when it came to selling.

Value in Fraudulent Pedigrees

Since simply having a pedigree increased the value of an animal, it soon became evident that by manufacturing bogus pedigrees people could run a lucrative business. The pedigree effects on markets quickly led to fraudulent uses of them in order to capitalize on the power they had over trade conditions. An overheated North American heavy horse trade in Clydesdales, Shires, and Percherons, late in the nineteenth century, encouraged the widespread problem of fraudulent horse dealers using false pedigrees. The American devotion to pedigrees as a guarantee of quality worked well with the ambitions of some horsemen who found they could dupe American farmers by providing false papers for crossbreds.[12] Dishonest stallion companies formed and encouraged that pattern. Dealers set up the companies and "peddled" poor stallions with bogus pedigrees.[13] Legitimate purebreds could be hard to separate from bogus purebreds. This situation, of course, undermined the position of horsemen owning males qualified for genuine pedigrees, and initiated the interest of purebred owners in some form of regulation over stallions taken out to public stud.

Purebred breeders with valid purebreds tried to defend their markets by using pedigrees as certificates of legitimacy against fraudulent or illegal activity. A movement for stallion licensing via enrolment and inspection arose from these pressures and relied on genuine pedigrees to regulate ethical trade in horses. What is particularly interesting about the stallion legislation and licensing story, however, is the fact that documentation around it provides much information on important matters unrelated to the bogus pedigree problem, namely matters involving an appreciation of how heredity worked, what connection purebred breeding had to quality, the role that pedigrees played either in markets or as guarantees of improvement, and the role of the state in breeding. The issue of fraudulent pedigrees, then, provides rich documentation on subjects normally either somewhat hidden or else so entangled with each other that it is hard to make sense of them.

An important background aspect to evolving North American stallion regulations and conflicts over the movement resulted from attitudes towards heredity which arose from the efforts of the 1888–9 British Royal Commission on Horse Breeding to define what made a stallion superior for breeding purposes.[14] The government's concern was primarily with horse improvement within Britain. Clearly the commissioners saw purebred breeding as an aspect of quality, but they believed that was only part of the story.[15] Much of their discussion centred on the problem of heredity itself. What caused horses to have weak legs and poor breathing, but, more importantly, could defects like these be inherited? Were these issues actually more serious than purebred status when it came to using a stallion at stud?[16] With these questions in mind, the commissioners turned to the Royal College of Veterinary Surgeons and asked it to identify hereditary defects, described as various aspects of "unsoundness" (skeletal or muscular problems).[17] The College sent the commissioners a list of defects thought to qualify as such, even though there was no consensus among vets as to what could be termed hereditary unsoundess.[18] The commission presented the list, dealing with the defects separately, to witnesses (all of whom were either veterinarians or horse breeders) at its 1889 hearings.

The confusion that arose from the complicated discussions that took place at the 1889 hearings[19] did not stop horsemen everywhere, after the release of an enormous report in 1890 that in fact concluded nothing, from believing that experts had answered the problem of heredity and unsoundness. While the report clearly suggested that purebred breeding and freedom from defects were both qualities of superior horses, it did not resolve an important dichotomy: how was one interconnected with the other? Regardless, the 1890 report laid the foundations for how stallion legislation would evolve over the next thirty years in many anglophone countries.[20] Quality, purebred breeding, and the genetic inheritance of certain characteristics would all be issues addressed by North American laws which licensed stallions to stand at public stud.[21] By the time the Commission released its 1890 report, owners of purebred stallions in North America, who made their living from the horses' stud fees, had faced such serious challenges to their business activities as a result of fraudulent activity that they had already taken some action. Pressure by purebred owners for state certification of purebred status in order to counteract bogus pedigrees resulted in the Illinois License Law for Stallions of 1887.[22] By 1890, then, the groundwork had been laid for confrontation and for discussion over what quality meant in horses, regardless of fraudulent activity. Structures were also in place to support an ongoing contentious movement designed to regulate breeding stallions.

The Illinois act initiated what would be a rising swell of voices against legislation that supported the interests of purebred breeders on the basis of pedigrees. By using pedigrees to designate stallions as purebred or crossbred under the act, even though enlisting the horses was voluntary (but for a fee), the designation aroused considerable concern. By dividing horses into purebreds and grades, the act seemed to encourage the idea, in the minds of ordinary horsemen, that purebreds were not just separate but also superior. These people did not see the fraudulent activity of some horse traders as the driver behind the legislation: for them the act pitted good crossbreds against purebreds. The apparent trend aroused antipathy from general horsemen. Furthermore, the act initiated a move towards state interference in breeding, a fact which struck many people as ominous for the future. Repeal the law and put everyone on the same footing, was a common cry, namely protection for nobody.[23] New templates for stallion acts followed first in Canada and then the United States, which further inflamed the situation over the years.

The 1903 legislation of the Northwest Territories in Canada introduced compulsory enrolment.[24] General reactions to future laws designed under that template matched those prevalent since the 1880s: opposition to purebred stallion support and to incursion on personal rights.[25] In 1906 a Wisconsin act, modelled on the legislation of the Northwest Territories, brought in an entirely new element to stallion regulation, namely enforced stallion categorization on the basis of soundness.[26] All stallions standing for public service in that state after 1906 were classified as to their purebred versus grade status and their level of quality within that status, as well as their relative soundness.[27] Quality of type and freedom from unsoundness, however, were only authorized by owners. Defects defined as unsoundness closely followed those on the list presented to the British Horse Commission in 1889. Its 1890 report had served as a reference point in the act's description of what constituted proven, hereditary unsoundness.[28] The Wisconsin legislation deviated, however, from the report by more openly equating purebred breeding with freedom from defects. When other states adopted the Wisconsin regulations, which encouraged government support for the concept that purebreds did not have hereditary defects, opposition became more widespread and more complicated. While the act triggered reactions commonly seen since the 1880s – Shouldn't people be allowed to breed as they wished? What about the erosion of personal liberty, important in a democratic country? Did experts know more than practical men?[29] Why consider purebreds innately superior to crossbreds? – the newly introduced question of health and soundness in relation to heredity introduced important controversy throughout North America.

The problem of defects in relation to purebred breeding, to pedigrees as a guarantee of either quality or freedom from inherited faults, now came to the forefront in many discussions taking place among horsemen. The differences of opinion between purebred breeders and general breeders were sharp. Many horsemen did not accept the purebred breeders' conviction that purebred breeding meant freedom from defects, and therefore that pedigrees acted as a guarantee. The linkage, its meaning and veracity, stimulated much discussion in the farm press. Many questions were raised, the following serving as examples. What was more important to the maintenance of quality: purebred breeding or soundness? Was a sound grade inferior to an unsound purebred? Why control stallions and not mares? How did one deal with the fact that soundness did not last a lifetime in horses, or at least could not be guaranteed to do so? Concepts concerning quality, soundness, and heredity became hopelessly entangled with another issue addressed by the act, namely validation of legitimate pedigrees in the face of bogus pedigrees. Purebred breeders continued to argue that the law protected farmers by guaranteeing the animal to be what it was stated to be, and it protected the stallion owner (through a lien on the resulting foal) by ensuring that fees would be paid (which, in turn, would defray the expense of buying good stallions). The fraudulent activity of horsemen trading in false pedigrees had, in fact, played into the hands of purebred breeders, who could legitimately argue that the public should be protected from this form of dishonesty.[30]

Pedigrees as a Marketing Cartel

A shift in purebred breeder objectives evolved after 1900 in both Canada and the United States, although the fraudulent pedigree issue played a role in masking that reality. Breeders might argue that the bogus pedigree problem drove their concern with regulation, but in fact they had become concerned more with expanding their market share than with simply protecting it. It was a short step to utilizing pedigrees not only to separate legitimate pedigrees from bogus ones but also to distinguish purebreds from crossbreds for trade purposes. Breeders devised a plan to expand their markets on the basis of dividing the horse population into animals with pedigrees and animals without. Pedigrees then became employed to create a marketing cartel against crossbred stock by enhancing the position of purebred breeders in relation to those who did not breed under the purebred structure. Breeder argument centred on the idea that purebred breeding was essential for the production of quality animals, and therefore that an extension of their interests was justifiable. After 1900 they were able to put forward their message effectively because they were better organized. The Ontario situation provides a particularly good example of these trends, because the problems of fraudulent pedigrees and dishonest stallion syndicates were less serious in that location than in either western Canada or the United States. Therefore the underlying motivation behind breeder interest in stallion regulation was more obvious in Ontario. Discussions that took place between horsemen and purebred breeders, in relation to the development of a marketing cartel with state blessing, elucidate even more clearly the differing positions each group held on the important issues that had emerged in earlier legislation.

Not only do confused attitudes that contemporaries held about the nature of heredity emerge in considerable detail in documentation around the issue in Ontario, but clarification of the fact that dichotomies ran through them also becomes evident. Documentation makes it clear too that the ongoing drive of purebred breeders to expand their markets over those for crossbreds or grades most emphatically could override their interest in breeding superior stock. Perhaps most important of all, however, documentation explains the basis for opinions and views of non-purebred breeders; this is very significant because their reasoning often stood in stark contrast to that of purebred breeders, government, and agricultural experts.

Much of the primary source material that we have today on either purebred breeding or attitudes to pedigrees is generated by purebred breeders, making it difficult to clarify in any detail how and why general livestock breeder convictions differed. Horsemen spoke up, and in doing so made evident what their views were concerning how heredity worked and in relation to general purebred and crossbred controversies. Because non-purebred breeders made up the vast majority of the population dealing with the animals, information on what they thought is highly significant to this story. Census data shows that at no time did purebreds dominate any animal population in either the United States or Canada, indicating clearly that ordinary breeders did not flock to the purebred system.[31] They were heartily criticized over the years for not doing so, and for being so short-sighted as to their welfare.

One Canadian purebred breeder, for example, argued in 1900 that purebred animals "must be bought and used by every farmer before Canadian agriculture will be as profitable as it should be."[32] The expense of purebred stock, relative to crossbreds, certainly played a role in farmers' avoidance of purebred stock, but it would appear that there were considerable intellectual differences between the animal breeding groups as well. Farmers did not see the triangle of quality, purity, and pedigree, for example, the same way that purebred breeders did. Farmers understood the process of heredity itself differently (and in many ways more correctly). Ordinary horsemen had clear opinions regarding breeding methodology, views on state interference in breeding decisions, attitudes towards heredity itself and the role of experience in the ability to breed properly, and conflicting convictions concerning the meaning of quality. Farm journal commentary and face-to-face discussions between ordinary and purebred breeders yield rich information about these reactions to the purebred industry.

Ontario purebred breeders began their crusade for market control by suggesting that, while the Wisconsin act of 1906 provided a good template for future Ontario legislation, it needed specific revisions. Only purebreds with recognized pedigrees should qualify for enrolment, and inspection should be both mandatory and government authorized. Purebred breeders, who connected unsoundness solely with grades, believed that certified purebreds would pass inspection; the issue of unsoundness would not affect them. Therefore it was safe to enforce government inspection for all stallions.[33] The general favouring of purebred breeding as improved breeding, an attitude prevalent in governments, meant that the desires of the breeders could not be simply dismissed out of hand. Increasingly strident and organized campaigns characterized the efforts of the newly formed Ontario Horse Breeders' Association after 1906 to force the government (which knew the farming public did not want such regulations) to enact legislation that essentially established a state-orchestrated marketing cartel on the basis of pedigrees.[34]

The Ontario minister of agriculture reacted by initiating an investigation into the matter. The minister divided Ontario into districts and sent two inspectors (often purebred breeders) to each in order to assess the quality of stallions serving at stud. At different locations within each district, public meetings were held in an attempt to ascertain what views general horsemen held with regard to enrolment and licensing and inspection for soundness. Reports seemed to indicate a favouring of both enrolment and inspection, but a closer read of statements reveals that most remarks made were not those of general farmers. The predominance of comments such as that enrolment should be limited to stallions with pedigrees (meaning those with legitimate registration papers) or that "scrub" (meaning mongrel) stallions should be kept off the road implied that the remarks were those of purebred breeders and also that the latter far outnumbered owners of grade stallions at the meetings.[35] A few investigators advised caution when trying to interpret the meaning behind these recurring statements. Being aware that purebred breeders dominated the meetings, they knew that many remarks did not necessarily indicate that horsemen in general favoured legislation.[36]

Within that framework, it is interesting to note the relatively few remarks made by grade stallion owners at the various public meetings. Observations could be particularly remarkable in light of the history of livestock genetics: namely, with respect to Bakewellian doctrine in the eighteenth century, the nature of purebred breeding in the nineteenth century, and the subsequent development of quantitative genetics in the mid-twentieth century. It was not uncommon at the 1906/7 meetings for horsemen owning grades or crossbreds to adhere to Bakewell's (and later quantitative genetic) theory regarding the value of the progeny test and the significance of females in breeding. Grade owners suggested that licensing stallions should be done on the basis of quality in foals produced by the stallion and also that it was equally important to license mares, because poor horses resulted from poor mares.[37] The survey revealed that the majority of stallions at public stud were purebred, but some of these animals could also be described as "scrubs" or "unfit" because of their unsoundness.[38] While breeders might want to equate soundness with purebreds, evidence from this survey clearly indicated that could not be done. The results of the investigation showed how confusing these attitudes, prevalent at the time throughout North America, were about the meaning of such words as "unfit" or "scrub" in relation to "unsoundness" or to purebred versus grade breeding.[39] The inquiry stimulated heated discussion in the farm press about the desirability of enforcing inspection and licensing by the enrolment of travelling stallions.[40] "Just where to draw the line in the granting or withholding of a license seems to be the stumbling block of this licensing plan," the *Farming World* noted.[41] Like many North Americans, the *Farmer's Advocate* worried about the right of government to interfere in stock breeding through regulation. Freedom for all, many argued: those who wanted grade horses had a right to get them, and those who wanted purebreds could have that too.[42] And what did the government know about breeding stallions anyway, one owner asked?[43]

The Ontario Horse Breeders' Association, after meeting to discuss the report of the 1906/7 investigation, decided on the following recommendations. Purebred registered stallions, having passed inspection, should be enrolled as Class 1. Grade horses, government inspected but only from good sires, should be allowed to enrol for three years as Class 2. Three inspectors should be appointed by the government for each district.[44] The association was prepared to accept some compromise with respect to enrolling grades. Purebred breeders believed grade numbers would be severely restricted because most would be disqualified for unsoundness. Furthermore, after three years, all grades (even acceptable ones) would be legislated off the road. Directors of the

Ontario Horse Breeders' Association, along with representatives of the Ontario government, which was willing to enact some purebred breeder requests, if not all, submitted the recommendations to horsemen across the province for discussion in 1908.[45] A detailed look at what was said at meetings shows how little was understood about heredity, the difficulties that arose from attempts to legislate improvement when no one could agree what improvement meant, and how conflicting were the definitions of "unfit" and "scrub" in relation to those for quality or soundness. It is also evident that purebred breeders often could not provide adequate answers to justifiable questions raised by farmers.

Pedigrees and their relationship to grading categories triggered considerable conversation. A horseman asked if the grade 1 and 2 system merely distinguished purebred from grade, and was told that was the case, though both classes had to have good conformation. Government representatives reiterated that registration by classification was intended simply to make it clear to a farmer whether a stallion was grade or purebred. A farmer responded: Why not just say registered and unregistered? The grading system implied quality superiority in purebreds, as far as farmers were concerned, not an effort to differentiate grades from purebreds. One claimed that he had a crossbred Shire/French Canadian, "as good a horse as ever was collared," which could trot thirty-six miles and could outwork his neighbour's pair of purebred Clydes. "Do not tie the farmers' hands; I do not think it is right," he added.[46] "I am not in sympathy with this resolution [to legislate on these issues]. It [creates] a monopoly of the Horse Breeders' Association," another concluded, "and we do not want that, there are a few men who want to monopolize the whole thing."[47] Farmers were aware that pedigrees always enhanced selling potential, and also that the actions of the government and breeders were intended to promote that trend.

The connection of unsoundness to heredity provoked considerable debate when horsemen questioned what reasons purebred breeders had for linking the two together. When a general farmer asked how, just because a horse was sound, you could say it was free of hereditary unsoundness, a purebred breeder answered that you had to know the stallion's ancestors. Another breeder contradicted this statement, saying a horse's ancestors did not determine hereditary soundness. The individual's status did. Farmers basically adhered to the following reasoning. Since breeders only wanted to identify and weed out those males that could perpetuate unsoundness, an unsound stallion that could not pass on his unsoundness should not be considered a problem from the breeding point of view. For horsemen, soundness and unsoundness were not by definition hereditary issues. (Modern veterinary opinion on the nature of horse heredity supports the contention that restriction of breeding stallions on the basis of various skeletal, muscular, respiratory, or neurological syndromes would not substantially reduce the problems in the general horse population.)[48] The question of quality as inherently lacking in grades and existing in purebreds was also raised. Legitimate purebreds were not by definition superior, many thought.

At the conclusion of the 1908 meetings, and in spite of the continuing evidence that many horsemen had serious concerns with what purebred stallion owners were trying to do, the Ontario Horse Breeders' Association pressed the government for legislation. Perhaps because the agenda of purebred breeders was clearly exposed at the 1908 meetings, where they faced questions from horsemen directly, the government hesitated for some time to take any action. In 1912 it finally passed the Ontario Stallion Enrolment Act, which compromised purebred breeder wishes to some extent: enrolment was enforced (purebred and grade stallions) but inspection was optional.[49] The *Advocate* canvassed opinions in 1913 on the new stallion act. No one was pleased: people thought it did either too much or too little.

Many purebred owners disliked the act because, by permitting grades to enrol, it put grades on the same level as purebreds.[50] Get the scrubs off the road.[51] Grade stallion owners argued that enrolment did not promote good breeding principles. The importance of progeny testing and the significance of mares in any breeding program, for example, often framed their reactions to the stallion act of 1912. After forty years' experience in breeding stallions, one grade owner stated in 1914 that inspection would not work because stallions should be judged by their progeny, not by inspection. Furthermore, the focus on stallions ignored the fact that the mare played an important role in the resulting foal. Stallion inspection was relatively ineffectual because so many mares were unsound. "What do you expect, apples off a thorn tree, or cranberries from a gooseberry bush?" Grade owners also argued that too much emphasis went to success in the show system: stallions winning prizes could not be deemed, as a result, to be good breeders.[52] Some purebreds should be described as scrubs, and grades should not be thought of necessarily as being scrubs.[53]

The Ontario Horse Breeders' Association pressed on to achieve what it had originally desired: compulsory inspection and the enrolment only of pedigreed purebreds.[54] The government capitulated. Effective August 1914, inspection would be compulsory.[55] Diseases (really malformations) considered not acceptable were the same as those presented in the 1890 report of the British Horse Commission.[56] By 1916, "no grade stallion of the scrub order, that having diseases or malformations mentioned in the regulations, shall be allowed to stand, travel, or be offered for service." By 1918, no grade stallion of any kind, even if free of unsoundness, would be allowed to breed.[57] The Ontario Horse Breeders' Association had finally got what it set out to achieve in 1906. Force, rather than encouragement, now characterized stallion legislation in Ontario. Stiffening the rigour of the act did nothing to decrease criticism of it, especially by grade stallion owners.[58] Even the *Advocate* continued to have mixed feelings about the act, because of the fundamental difficulty in legislating for quality, the unclear understanding of what constituted hereditary unsoundness, and the problem of force rather than encouragement over breeding. "In Ontario the grade stallion [was] being legislated out of business."[59] Not having a pedigree meant much-reduced monetary value.

The hot market for Clydes, Shires, and Percherons (more on this in the next chapter) had created problems within North America, which led to a movement in which the state would direct breeding. Pedigrees had served as a critical device in legislating how stallion service would proceed and, more importantly, designating which stallions were economically valuable and which were not. Pedigrees, then, were at the heart of the matter. While stallion legislation would not endure (the working horse market effectively collapsed with the rise of internal combustion engines), pedigrees and trade continued to be linked in the livestock market. The issue of having a pedigree versus not having a pedigree would persist in affecting trade in animals.

The Perfection Case: Purity by Pedigree in Herefords

By the 1970s, a purebred beef cattle revolution had completely altered the shape of the beef industry. The emphasis over decades on breeding for short, blocky cattle initiated the revolution, and at least partially resulted from decisions made by show judges about cattle phenotype.[60] Their collective views reflected theories put forward by agricultural colleges across the United States and Canada about what constituted quality in a beef animal.[61] Uniformity of judges' opinions concerning the style across many subsequent show ring events not only brought about pronounced breeding shifts within the purebred world but also shaped public opinion about desirable traits in commercial cattle. Show results were particularly influential on the general herds in the 1940s and 1950s, when purebreds probably exerted their greatest impact on commercial cattle, a trend that had begun around 1920.[62] By the 1950s it had become apparent that judges' support for short, blocky phenotypes had introduced a serious genetic defect producing not just small cattle but also dwarfism, an autosomal recessive defect. As early as the nineteenth century, dwarfism had been observed in cattle. The small Dexter breed had experienced the rise of a form of dwarfism known as "bull dog."

When a different type of dwarfism, known as "snorter," became evident in the mid-twentieth century within the dominant North American beef breeds of the time (namely Shorthorns, Hereford, and Angus), considerable support emerged for the conviction that selection practices and inbreeding, based on decisions of show judges, encouraged the rise of the recessive defect in the herds. It also seemed that the defective gene, when present heterozygously, changed the phenotypic appearance of an animal. Show judges claimed that they could visually recognize snorter carriers, for example, yet research suggested that they were right only 50 per cent of the time.[63] Phenotypic expression could not be relied on to accurately identify carriers.[64] Numerous studies, however, made it clear that carriers *as a group* were different from non-carriers *as a group*, by being shorter of leg and by maturing earlier (males particularly). Since these characteristics represented what show judges looked for, it seems clear that selection favoured carriers, which brought about the rise of defective snorter calves.[65] The problem seemed particularly severe in Herefords.[66] One 1956 survey estimated that there were about fifty thousand dwarf-producing Herefords in the United States, a problem that breeders, scientists, and the American Hereford Association attacked through pedigree analysis and breeding trials. Since carrier status was often difficult to determine (no DNA test existed), even lines thought to potentially involve carriers were completely destroyed. As a result, the defect was reduced to such a level (due to the elimination of much recessive/recessive inheritance in calves) that it virtually never appeared by 1970 in the Hereford breed.[67] But that did not lead to recovery of the breed's popularity. The demand for larger cattle was the death knell for even healthy short-statured cattle.

The dwarfism debacle not only played an important role in triggering the beef cattle importation revolution but also led to revisions in judges' opinions regarding desirable style in show animals. After 1960, taller and leaner stock became favoured, more in line with the size of larger Continental breeds like Simmental and Charolais. Judges' demands for ever larger sized animals continued unabated until the late 1980s. The frame scores of animals between the 1950s and 1990 demonstrate the dramatic shifts in style that judging brought about. (Frame score is a method of estimating relative skeletal size of adult cattle based on hip height. Frame scores vary from one to eleven.) Show cattle of the 1950s often had a frame score of less than one. By 1990 the frame score of show winners averaged ten or higher.[68] The drive for larger and leaner cattle forced Hereford breeders to change breeding aims. Their cattle could not compete either in the market place or in the show ring. At first breeders tried to recover by breeding for size within registered lines, but it proved difficult because of the narrowed genetic field available to them due to dwarfism and restrictive demands for pedigree purity. They became increasingly desperate. By the late 1970s, Hereford breeders had begun to introduce crossbreeding or breeding up in their programs, albeit in an underhanded manner within that registry environment which demanded purity.

In 1983 what turned out to be a remarkable bull was born within that environment. Named KLC RB3 Perfection, by the time he was three years old he had proven to be a sensation (particularly noteworthy for any of the British breeds) by being a show winner and sire of the tall, lean calves so desired by the new beef industry. He amassed a fortune for his owner, Dr Willard Keith, a wealthy hobbyist breeder. Rumblings were in the air, however, as other Hereford breeders became suspicious about the bull's ancestral background in relation to purity. Some argued that Perfection's registered Hereford dam, Bold Victriss 51, was in fact half red Holstein. Jealousy also seemed to play a role in the accusation because it was well known that top Hereford breeders were carefully introducing foreign genetics in order to increase the stature of their cattle, even if the matter was never publicly brought to light. Blood tests were conducted on Victress's full sister, Sis, to see if it could be proven that the two cows came from the same mother. (Victress had died in 1984 without having any blood test done on her.) There was no match, meaning no one could prove what animal had been Victriss's dam. On the basis of such evidence, in 1986 the authorities of the American Hereford Association and of the American Polled Hereford Association managed to convince the organizations to deregister both Perfection and all his descendants. The Canadian Hereford Association followed suit. By that time, semen sales had become huge, and each individual descendant of Perfection was believed to be worth $265,000. In Canada roughly 10 per cent of Hereford breeders relied on Perfection breeding. Clearly Perfection had proven to be of huge economic value, and non-pedigreeing him and his descendants would cause great hardship. The animals' value would be reduced to virtually nothing.[69]

There were two reactions. One was an attempt to form a new registry. Cattlemen ruined by deregistry of Perfection stock tried to form the International Hereford Organization in order to certify Perfection animals, and, as one article stated, to "declare the bull once more as purebred."[70] The other reaction proved to be more fruitful. Perfection's owner and those involved in marketing his semen brought nine lawsuits against the Hereford associations. The owners wanted $400 million in damages, and finally in 1989 the associations, in order to avoid such payments, capitulated without bringing the issue to court. They agreed to reinstate the pedigree status of the bull and of his progeny that had been conceived before August of 1989. Cattle with Perfection background, however, were to be stigmatized: the letter "L" was to go before their registration number. Furthermore, Keith was debarred from the organizations and ordered to breed no more Herefords. In many ways it was a Pyrrhic victory for those determined to demote Perfection, but on the other hand the bull's popularity was enormously diminished by the chain of events. The crisis of that allegiance to purity, pedigrees, and the connection of both to monetary worth faded into the background quickly, as breeders tried to forget the debacle. Then in 2012 the *Hereford World* published an article in which the two main drivers of deregistering Perfection and his stock were honoured for taking on rich investors who violated the mission statement of the American Hereford Association (the two associations had been forced to amalgamate over the issue), which was to preserve the purity of the breed, to enforce the keeping of herd book pedigree integrity.[71]

Breeders who had lived through the "Perfection" case were quick to react to the tone of the article. On the Internet Chat line *Hereford Talk*, a discussion took place which showed clearly that the general consensus of breeders was that Keith had been singled out for self-serving reasons which had nothing to do with purity. As one writer stated: "A doctor from back east who is a newbie ... smokes everyone in the [show] ring and people start grumbling." He did what everyone else was doing. He was made an example of. He wasn't old guard, not politically big, so the powerful men in the Hereford industry thought they could bust him and get rid of his cattle so they could win. "Perfection's owner and breeder was an easy target albeit a costly one – new guy, hobby breeder, didn't cover ... tracks well and [wasn't] with it enough to use something [an animal for breeding] that had a chance of not raising suspicion right off the bat."[72] Another breeder agreed. "Perfection's breeders and owners were not well connected with the leadership of the American Polled Hereford Association or the American Hereford Association and that made them easy targets. The owners may have had personal wealth but they had little power or influence with either association." This writer had heard direct rumours from others involved with the Perfection story that the bull was in fact crossbred. A person the writer knew had told a friend that "he knew Perfection was a crossbred and the reason blood tests didn't show him to be a crossbred was because breeders used red Holsteins to add size to the Herefords because differences in blood test types between Herefords and Holsteins wouldn't be detected by the then used test." When the writer confronted this person, the individual flatly denied saying anything about Perfection's purity.[73] Clearly the story around Perfection was clouded with many issues, most of which had nothing to do with purity but plenty to do with the power of pedigrees over monetary affairs and as a driver in the market. Non-pedigree status greatly curtailed both, regardless of quality.

Pedigrees: The Making of Crossbred Horses into "Breeds"

The fortunes of crossbred Arabian horse types over this period show the same marketing power of simply having a pedigree versus not having one. In the 1970s, Gene LaCroix Jr, a breeder and horseman deeply involved with the Arabian horse for years, saw that the ancient linkage of pedigrees to marketing could be used in other ways than as a tool to prove or provide evidence of purity, or even hereditary background. For him it presented an opportunity to increase the value of crossbred horses, with no need to define them as "pure," or even consistent as to phenotype. LaCroix believed that, by providing a popular type of existing crossbred horse, the American Saddlebred/Arabian, with a pedigree system, he could enhance the value of the animals and himself in the process. In 1981 he named the crossbreds National Show Horses (NSH), and in 1982 established an independent registry for them. In doing so he introduced new patterns to how the old triangle based on pedigree, breeding, and marketing worked: market factors drove pedigreeing; it was not a situation where pedigrees drove markets.

LaCroix set standards for entry into the new registry as loosely as possible. Purity was not an issue: pedigreeing simply meant "certifying" or accrediting a well-known system of crossbreeding. By amalgamating two breeds, LaCroix planned to form a crossbred breed. The National Show Horse Registry Board (which LaCroix established) nominated stallions from either breed to serve as foundation sires for foals eligible for pedigree status. National Show Horses could have as little as 25 per cent Arabian blood, or as much as 99 per cent.[74] (It was assumed that the dam would be some variation of Arabian or Saddlebred.) At the National Arabian Horse Show of 1982, where many animals carrying Saddlebred blood were eligible for entry as Half-Arabians, the new registry offered prize money to horses with National Show Horse Registry (NSHR) pedigrees. Entries in the NSHR book rose immediately from 90 to 400. Within a year of operation, the registry had issued 1400 pedigrees and had listed 190 nominated stallions. Soon exhibitions for NSHR horses were held, and, by 1985, fully orchestrated sales were also run – both of which enhanced the monetary value of the animals.[75] By operating an open stud book with regulations designed to protect quality and type, and by providing marketing devices such as show and sale operations, LaCroix organized and formalized breeding efforts already in existence and then capitalized on the increased marketability of the resulting horses, as did his fellow breeders. Shortly after 2000, the American Saddlebred introduced LaCroix to another horse which interested him in exploring a new pedigreed, crossbred project. Pedigrees, again, would play a critical role in the "creation" of a breed.

LaCroix devised a way of combining the genetics of the Dutch Warmblood and the Arabian and of using the European culture of inspection and licensing as a method of setting standards for entry into an open stud book. In effect he decided that by combining the purebred breeding method with breeding under a standardbred system designed to assess utility or athletic ability, he could attract people to a different way of certifying quality in a horse. The complicated cultural interplay in this endeavour must be seen within the framework of certain standardbred breeding systems as opposed to purebred breeding, how and where warmbloods developed, and the historical background of the Dutch Warmblood itself. Standardbred breeding was not focused, as chicken breeding had been, on beauty points. Standardbred breeding of horses was a system designed to recognize quality and type under performance testing. Animals were required to meet certain standards such as the ability to run, to undergo certain athletic exercises, and endurance requirements. Success in performance testing was the basis for recording in registries. Unlike purebred breeding, which rests solely on the foundation of genealogical background, standardbred breeding rests on the idea that individual animals had to display certain characteristics and prove through testing that they possessed them.

The classic animal that developed under standardbred breeding is the Standardbred trotting horse, pedigreed in the early days on the basis of the ability to trot a certain distance at a certain speed.[76] Warmbloods are horses bred and developed under a similar system which required some proof of worth via testing before an animal could be pedigreed. Such horses have an ancient European lineage and resulted from various crosses of so-called cold blood from the heavy draft types or breeds on the so-called hot blood of the Arabian, Thoroughbred, Hackney, Saddlebred, or Morgan. Warmbloods are not "breeds" the same way that cold and hot blood breeds are, in that they are not pedigreed solely on the basis of genealogy. They have registry systems that maintain open stud books, and therefore profit from hybrid vigour that comes with outcrosses. Warmbloods reflect breeding strategies resting on the belief that quality in individual animals should be evaluated by inspection and subsequently licensed. Pedigrees on the basis of ancestry offered no such qualification. Most types originated in central Europe. They were all originally working animals, designed to meet agricultural needs, provide transportation for rural people, or supply rulers with remounts for the army. The breeding methods applied to the warmbloods (open registries, emphasis on type, and athletic ability standards set by inspection and performance testing) reintroduced North Americans to horse breeding patterns that had been prevalent before the advent of purebred breeding.

The Dutch Warmblood, which would become linked to the Arabian in the United States, was derived in the Netherlands from various crosses of French, German, and English horses on local animals. Over the years, two distinct types of the Dutch Warmblood appeared: the more active animal from Gelderland, and one from Groningen. The varieties were freely interbred with each other and were triple purpose in nature until the 1960s. A third one, a harness horse known as a Tuigpaard, or the Dutch Harness Horse, was invented in the 1970s from Dutch Warmbloods and the addition of Hackney blood. The Tuigpaard resulted from an attempt to produce a high-stepping, elegant show animal that could be either driven or ridden. A stud book for the Dutch Warmblood had been set up in 1970 (several local and regional books for the Gelderlander and Groninger existed before that time) and became the Koninklijk Warmbloed Paardenstamboek Nederland, or the KWPN Studbook in 1988.[77] The three separate horse variations qualify as Dutch Warmbloods: the riding horse (largest section), the Gelders horse (also generally ridden), and the Dutch Harness Horse.

To be recorded in this stud book, all horses must undergo rigid inspection, called keuring, which generally speaking starts at the age of three years. Mares are evaluated for conformation and movement, but are subsequently further ranked in accordance with the quality of the foals they produce. Inspection and testing of stallions is more stringent than that of mares. Every year young stallions must undergo a seventy-day test, where conformation, paces, and attitude are assessed. If the stallions meet certain standards, they are classified as either "keur" (choice) or at a higher level as "preferent" (preferred).[78] In 1983 the KWPN set up the North American Department, called the NA/WPN, for the Dutch Warmblood in the United States, to promote the horse in that country. The name of the NA/WPN was changed to the Dutch

Warmblood Studbook of North America in 1997. The riding type used for jumping and dressage maintained the most popularity in the United States. The Dutch Harness Horse was relatively unknown before 2000, but after that it burst onto the scene through the work of LaCroix.[79]

In 1999 an American breeder of Saddlebreds, Clarke Vestry, came in contact with a Dutch breeder of Dutch Harness Horses, Marcel Ritsma. The result was a partnership and the import in the year 2000 of several Dutch Harness Horses to La Grange, Kentucky, where Vestry lived and which was also the home of LaCroix. By the end of 2000, between seventy-five and one hundred Dutch Harness Horses had been exported to the United States. The KWPN reacted quickly to this rapid growth in sales by setting up systems for inspection of Dutch Harness Horses specifically for recording purposes in North America. The first keuring of Dutch Harness Horses (or DHH) in North America took place under the Dutch authorities in the summer of 2001 in Kentucky. The European open registry, with its contingent regulations regarding licensing, came with the breed to North America.

LaCroix recognized quickly that a marketing potential existed in the promotion of a crossbred Dutch Harness Horse/Arabian through a pedigree system. Furthermore, he himself owned and promoted a DHH keur-approved stallion.[80] Using a recording system designed to resemble the Dutch keuring method, LaCroix added another new dimension to his scheme.[81] He set up what was known as the Renai Registry and hoped to show the Arabian horse world not just the value of the new warmbloods in the breeding of show horses but also the advantages offered by the breeding culture that produced them. As he explained:

> For long-term success, a responsible horse breed organization must protect, perpetuate and constantly improve the breed it governs. Leadership must establish clear standards of excellence. Conformation, movement and athletic function must be absolute prerequisite[s] to the achievement of these standards. In some of the pure breeds of horses today, particularly the Arabian, these qualities have been compromised in favor of "breed type" or "fashion" and their popularity significantly diminished. This is not fair to the integrity of these fine breeds, nor to the breeders, owners, and trainers that aspire to realize their maximum potential. Until now there has been no choice or better alternatives for those wishing to say loyal to their breed.[82]

LaCroix organized a system for approval and licensing of stallions within three divisions of the Renai Registry. Division A recorded stallions of various breeds that had been inspected and approved under conditions that resembled the keuring of the DHH. These stallions were to be foundation sires of what would be known as the Renai Horse. Division B registered pure Arabian stallions, also inspected but only after 2004, and these were labelled Renaissance Arabians. Division C listed stallions belonging to all show breeds, including the NSH, and even admitted qualified "crossbreds" or grades.[83] LaCroix also started orchestrating shows and sales in 2002 for the developing Renai "breed" and for Renai registered horses.[84] While his Renai horse would not endure, LaCroix believed that he had had a particularly visionary idea when it came to the Renai horse registry, as he explained in 2008, about the time that the registry folded.[85] LaCroix stated: "With the Renai Horse Registry, probably the best but most misunderstood concept I ever developed, the goal was to bring all Saddle Seat oriented breeds together by allowing breeders to breed for this specific performance [show gaits] without limitation to breed purity."[86]

At the same time that LaCroix was promoting the DHH as a show horse, its crossing on the Arabian for improvement of the Arabian as a high-gaited horse, and Dutch keuring for pedigree purposes, he attacked systems in place for the purebred Arabian, namely the structure of shows and correspondingly the lack of accepted breed standards designed to define beauty in the horses.[87] LaCroix seemed to be advocating an approach which supported a phenotypic point system like that used to evaluate exhibition chickens or the show quality of purebred dogs. Many Arabian horse breeders were as disenchanted as LaCroix with the show situation, and especially its relationship to breeding practices, as letters to the *Arabian Horse World* make clear.[88] Breeders tended to identify the main problem in the Arabian horse community, however, not so much as the lack of a structured point system but rather as the general infiltration of crossbreeding into the Arabian, especially the use of Saddlebred blood and the resulting effect that had on Arabian shows. The increased emphasis on the breeding of Saddlebred/Arabians, which entered shows as Half-Arabians, made many people believe the purebred Arabian was being undermined. They saw the phenomenon largely as the outcome of LaCroix's work over the previous thirty years. Purity, not crossbreeding, defined quality and also type, these breeders argued, in their adherence to the purebred outlook and the ancient view that Arabians were the original and the best of improved horses. A breeder with well over fifty years experience with Arabians and half-Arabians explained:

> I always [bred half-Arabians] so that Arabian blood could improve the other breed involved. I don't believe there is another breed on earth that

can improve the purebred Arabian. I think the alternative is to choose another breed if you don't like the purebred Arabian for some inexplicable reason. I love other breeds. Thoroughbreds bred for conformation and jumping I think are spectacular. They can sometimes be improved on with Arabian blood. Some of the large European breeds such as the Trakehner and Dutch Warmblood are magnificent beasts. They can be improved by Arabian blood and indeed it is frequently used. Using those breeds to produce something for us is totally non-productive because we don't get a better Arabian nor do we get anything as good for its purpose as the other breed involved. I love to see a spectacular Saddlebred, but the Half-Arabian version is just short of ridiculous in comparison.[89]

Many Arabian breeders agreed with this point of view. One stated: "The Half-Arabians certainly have their place, but it is not sharing the stage with the breed that made their existence possible ... [I have seen] many Half-Arabians looking, and often times performing like Saddlebreds. If I wanted to see that I would [go] to a Saddlebred show." Another letter to the *Arabian Horse World* added: "We find the promotion of the Half-Arabian at the expense of the purebred the most distressing trend."[90] One correspondent to the journal suggested that its name be changed to the *Half-Saddlebred World*. (The editor of the journal took exception, stating that the Arabian produced beautiful crosses.)[91] The Renai horse might not have taken hold, but the National Show Horse would endure and became virtually a breed in its own right. Considerable modification of the original standards, more in line with unity of phenotype, so typical of "pure" breeds, had developed by 2019.[92] Other half-Arabians of many varieties also endured and, in fact, have always been popular: Anglo Arabians (Thoroughbred Arabian crosses) and Pinto Arabians, to name a few.

While clearly LaCroix's work was controversial and also went against the mainstream of breeding with "purity" in mind, nothing could indicate more forcefully how important pedigrees were when it came to establishing a "breed." Attitudes to selection, namely what genetics would be worked with, and even the purebred system, which demanded uniformity of phenotype, did not initiate the demarcation of either "breed" or market worth. Pedigrees did. But while a registry and its recording of pedigrees might establish a group of animals as a "breed," some phenotypic uniformity would ultimately be essential for the continuing recognition of that group as a "breed." The demise of the Renai horse could, for example, have related to the completely open breed concept used for registry purposes, a cultural idea better received in Europe, and historically related to Warmbloods, than in the United

States. The fluidity of phenotype as a result of entry requirements seemed in this case to cancel the benefits that pedigreeing offered. People could not identify the selected group as a breed, and as a result stopped recording in the Renai Horse Registry. Pedigrees might have established the National Show Horse as a "breed," but its continuation seemed largely to rest on the development of great uniformity as to phenotype and a breed standard as to appearance.

Pedigrees clearly dictated relative value in animals, and even came to define the meaning of "breed." Their larger impact, however, came from the way they directed both breeding itself and the functioning of the international market; both are subjects of the next chapter.

Chapter Eight

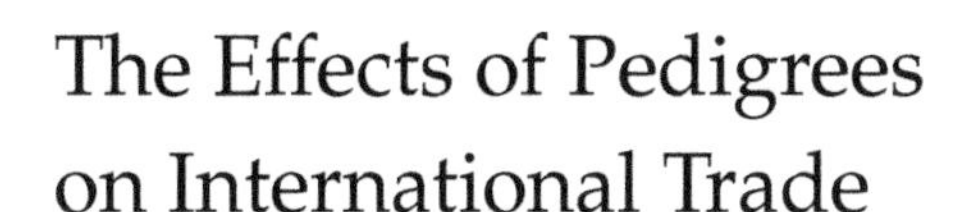

The Effects of Pedigrees on International Trade

An important dimension of the pedigree and trade story is the effect that the manipulation of pedigree standards could have on international markets. In this chapter I assess pedigree and trade regulations in the international market and how developments affected both the animals and their breeders from the nineteenth century to the twenty-first. Central to much of this narrative was the situation in the United States, both as to breeder views and the role of the state. The first part of the chapter looks at the international picture over the late nineteenth century, when various American breeder associations, together with the US government, controlled importation on the basis of pedigree standards. The second part reviews the international trade when American associations alone regulated standards for entry. Regardless of the US government's declining involvement, it will be clear that "purebredness" in all countries continued to reflect the influence of breeder positions in the United States. The third part of the chapter assesses a particular world trade situation by focusing on the work of an international breeder organization formed in the latter half of the twentieth century. The World Arabian Horse Organization (WAHO) set pedigree standards which directed global trade in Arabian horses into the twenty-first century. While the United States was only one member nation in this organization, that country played an important role in how WAHO functioned, and, as a result, how both breeding and marketing patterns developed around the world.

The historic notion that pedigrees should guide tariff-related trade between nations had been laid down as early as the end of the eighteenth century, with the advent of pedigrees for the Thoroughbred horse. All horses with General Stud Book (GSB) papers could move duty free between countries, because pedigrees in the GSB were believed to guarantee animal quality. By the mid-nineteenth century, numerous registry systems for other livestock breeds existed, thereby complicating the situation. Furthermore, when pedigree standards in herd books for a specific breed differed across nations, as had become the case by the late nineteenth century, assessing duty-free status became problematic. The dilemma of competing standards would be magnified when classic attitudes to pedigrees in European countries came to contrast sharply with those held in North America. The British and continental Europeans always held a more relaxed view towards both standards and even recording than did North Americans. Because animals of a certain type or breed were ubiquitous in the lands where they originated, many British and European people did not see a need to separate certain individuals from others via pedigrees. The circumstances were different in countries where the animals were rare and therefore exotic. Importing nations like Canada and the United States saw standards for entry to herd books as certification of the animal's imported genetic base. Commonly, pedigreeing in importing countries rested on one of two approaches to classifying legitimacy. The first was defined as the four cross system, which meant a breeding up from local animals and crossing with purebred registered animals over four generations. The other was described as a closed book attitude. Under a closed book system, only animals with purebred registered parents could be pedigreed. In effect the closed technique called for the highest possible level of imported genetics in an animal, and allowed for no breeding up.[1]

When it became evident to North Americans that, by manipulating standards between the four cross and closed book systems, they could regulate tariffs and therefore orchestrate markets, international trade in purebred livestock took on new characteristics, especially after breeders began to better organize themselves to achieve these ends.[2] The concurrent involvement of the American government in pedigree issues through legislation (culminating in the 1897 Dingley tariff bill) complicated the situation. Regulations of the 1913 American Underwood tariff bill brought change to the trade in purebred stock. The bill allowed all animals into the United States duty free, but it also initiated a permanent shift in American government attitudes to purebred breeding. After 1913, being purebred implied no special status as far as federal tariffs or involvement was concerned. Government would, as a result, no longer play a role in pedigree maintenance, standards, and importation patterns.[3] Over the years, tariffs on livestock would be reinstated at different times (particularly significant for cattle in the 1920s), and stock could even be denied entry, as was the case with the BSE, or mad cow disease, crisis in the twenty-first century. However, under these conditions, purebred breeding did not put animals into a different and special category. As far as the American government was concerned, all animals would be allowed in either duty free or subject to tariff, depending on what regulations were in place at the time. The breeders alone would regulate the meaning of purebred status, and did so through standards.

Pedigrees: Shorthorns and Ayrshires in Canadian-American Trade, 1880–1910

A review of the purebred trade between Canada and the United States in two breeds of cattle serves as one example of the way pedigree standards, breeders, and government came to influence the shape of a North American cross-border international trade by the late nineteenth century. The trade introduces a fundamental point: the outlook of the American associations and the American government together on pedigree matters stipulated how the international market would operate. The affairs of Shorthorn and Ayrshire breeders in Canada illustrate how people and cattle were affected by changing attitudes of American breeders and the United States government.

In 1876, Shorthorn breeders in the United States organized themselves into the American Shorthorn Breeders' Association in order to take control of standards, which at the time were administered by owners of three separate registry books. The books allowed the recording of animals under the four cross system. The breeders managed first to change the standards of Lewis Allen's American Short-Horn Book (the largest registry and the oldest) to the closed system only.[4] The move of American breeders over the 1870s to enforce the closed book system for all recording of Shorthorns in the United States created a difficult situation in Canada. The single registry for Shorthorns in the country, the Canada Short Horn Herd Book, had been maintained since 1867 by the Ontario government on the basis of the four cross system (cattle arising exclusively from imports, of course, qualified for entry as well). Canadian standards simply shut down many American markets for pedigreed Canadian animals.[5]

Prominent Canadian breeders adapted to American pressure for change by registering animals that met the criteria for a closed system pedigree in one of the American books, as revealed at the Ontario Agricultural Commission's hearings. John Clay, manager of the Bow Park breeding farm, explained: "The defect in the Canadian Herd Book is that it admits animals that have only four crosses, while an animal cannot be registered in the American Herd Book unless it can trace its pedigree to ... imported [ancestors]. The result is that the Canadian

Herd Book has not that standing among Shorthorn men that the American has."[6]

John Miller, another important breeder and importer, pointed out that the issue of accurately kept records versus spurious ones was equally important. "As far as I know," he stated, "the Canadian Herd Book is authentic" and "contains an honest record of the pedigrees ... A great many of the pedigrees in the American Herd Book have been disputed and found out to be wrong."[7] Miller still sold successfully into the United States on the basis of pedigrees recorded in the Canada Short Horn Herd Book and argued that an American buyer could find stock descended entirely from imported animals in the Canadian registry. It was a question of choice. Miller would soon find, however, that the climate in the United States concerning standards, as much as apprehension over spurious pedigrees, would change how the international market worked. Any herd book that allowed registration under four crosses would soon be unacceptable in the United States.

By 1880 American breeders were in favour of only recognizing foreign pedigrees from a book which recorded animals solely on the basis of the closed standards.[8] Canadian breeders reacted to the rising emphasis on the closed book by forming a Shorthorn breeder association in 1882. The new association planned to force the Ontario government (which maintained the only Canadian Shorthorn registry) to drop the recording of cattle under the four cross system and to establish a single closed registry system. It took four years for them to convince the Ontario government of the need for such a book.[9] It soon became obvious, however, that some important animals would not qualify for pedigrees under the new system. Distressing information arose out of discussions which showed that many of the best Shorthorns in Canada traced to a bull named Roger, who *might* have descended from non-pedigreed 1817 Shorthorn imports into Kentucky. Reluctantly, breeders decided that Shorthorns tracing to Roger should not qualify for the new Dominion Shorthorn Herd Book, because all animals eligible for pedigrees had to trace to imported stock registered in the British Shorthorn Coates's Herd Book.

The decision to drop Roger and his descendants and abolish any recording under the four cross system wiped out some farmers. Having no pedigree status, therefore not defined as "purebreds," their cattle lost a large part of their monetary worth. Some farm operations completely changed over the late 1880s and 1890s, when breeders could no longer designate their Shorthorn herds as purebred. A clear example of how significant these pedigree changes could be to a working farm can be seen in reports made to the government in 1886 and 1887 on the operations of an Ontario farm known as Balsam Lodge. In 1886, John Freeman and Thomas Shaw reported that Mr Fothergill, who owned Balsam Farm, maintained high-quality beef Shorthorns, having "deep heavy bodies on short limbs of medium bone, and possess[ing] much of the wealth of substance so eagerly sought for by Short Horn breeders today." By 1887 the situation was entirely different: "[In 1886] one of the principal products of the farm was beef; [in 1887] it is milk." Freeman and Shaw elaborated as follows:

> Owing to the recent change of standard adopted by the Dominion Short Horn Breeder's [*sic*] Association the major portion of the entire herd was cut off from the registry, so that Mr. Fothergill was necessitated to relay the foundation of another herd or go out of business. He chose the latter alternative, and has replaced those stately beauties with a herd of grade dairy cows whose principal mission is to furnish milk in large quantity ... The change just referred to necessitates some variation in the methods of tillage, but less of this than in the varieties of feed grown.[10]

By the late 1880s, Shorthorn breeders in Canada felt assured that their interests had been preserved by the move to make their standards match those of the United States, but after 1890 that increasingly appeared not to be the case. In 1897 the Dingley tariff led to future legislative action that would reinforce a position adhered to by American breeders, namely forced recording in the American registry before pedigree status, and therefore duty-free entry, could be granted. In 1906 the Bureau of Animal Industry (BAI) order 136 (which was authorized by the United States Department of Agriculture through directions from the Treasury Department under the Dingley tariff) instructed that all imported purebred animals had to be registered in the American books to obtain duty-free status and to be recognized as purebred in the United States.[11] Shorthorn breeders had already restricted entry by initiating their own form of protectionism: they charged non-American breeders a $100 fee to register animals in their herd book, a stipulation they continued to impose after the 1906 regulations were in place. Canadian breeders recognized the fee as being a tariff or tax imposed solely by the breed association, albeit with the blessing of the American government.[12] Government action gave legislative authority to the regulations of the American Shorthorn Association. The Canadians retaliated by asking their government to restrict American duty-free entry of Shorthorns not registered in the Canadian book.[13] The passing of the

Underwood bill drastically changed the picture, effectively undermining the BAI's authority over the American registration of the purebred breeds.[14]

Canadian Ayrshire cattle breeders went through similar attempts to adjust to American pedigree standards in order to maintain market connections. In the 1870s, the breeders had organized themselves in two associations, one in Quebec and one in Ontario, but in 1880 no herd books, established on the basis of agreed-upon standards with records of animals registered to those standards, existed in the breed.[15] A livestock registrar had been established as early as 1854 by the Ontario government to print pedigrees for "thoroughbred animals" on the basis of owner records, but no Ayrshires were registered under that system before 1872. Imported stock might have pedigrees from their country of origin (generally speaking, Scotland), which served as a base for private records. In some cases, however, imported Ayrshires were simply cows that had won at milking shows in the region of Ayrshire, Scotland, and did not have pedigrees.[16]

Troubles with the American market made Ayrshire breeders organize themselves and develop a pedigreeing system more systematically, with clear standards for entry into a herd book. By amalgamating breed associations in Quebec and Ontario, and enforcing a closed pedigree system for a new united herd book (both achieved by 1898), they hoped they could maintain markets in the United States.[17] The value of certain animals had to be sacrificed along the way, however, in order to achieve reciprocity in pedigree recognition. Difficulties had emerged over the pedigree of a certain cow named Lady of the Lake (calved in 1859). Americans did not see Lady of the Lake (and therefore her descendants) as eligible for a closed herd book. One descendant in particular, a bull named Bonnie Scotland, had been important to Quebec breeders. Like the Shorthorn bull Roger, Bonnie Scotland and his progeny had to be removed in order for Americans to accept Canadian Ayrshires.[18]

The new Canadian Ayrshire Association was determined to make its standards identical to those of the United States, meaning a closed herd book and agreement on all pedigrees. Many Ayrshire breeders found their financial situation greatly changed by the removal of the cow and her descendant, Bonnie Scotland. Like their Shorthorn counterparts, Ayrshire breeders would find that American markets were not guaranteed by these adjustments. The regulations set up through the Dingley tariff affected Ayrshire affairs as much as they did Shorthorns. Pedigrees, in effect, had come to define the import status of animals with respect to whether free trade prevailed or did not; and furthermore the recording of long-dead individual animals within a registry had the power to undermine years of breeding: the past could haunt the present (and future) when standards for entry were changed.

Pedigrees: Clydesdale and Shire Horses in the Transatlantic Trade, 1880–1910

By the late nineteenth century, pedigree standards not only controlled how the international trade in animals of the same breed worked but also led to the moulding of existing breed phenotypes and the creation of new breeds. A particularly good example of the breeding, and therefore moulding, pattern arising from American manipulation of pedigree standards can be seen in the dynamics of the heavy horse world of the late nineteenth century. Heavy horse types were relatively new in the American equine scene in 1880 (the *Breeder's Gazette* stated that American farmers knew little about the truly heavy horses before 1872)[19] when the issue of pedigrees, standards, and import regulations began to play such an important role in the international livestock trade. Breeding methods applied to the Clydesdale and the Shire would be guided by standards set in relation to American importation. American ideas concerning pedigree standards and "purity" first transformed these heavy horse types into "purebreds" or breeds, and subsequently changed their phenotype.[20]

Both the Clyde and the Shire had developed from the merging of local stock from various backgrounds. Purity of genealogy played no role in how breeding evolved. The Clydesdale type, like the English Shire type, resulted from late eighteenth-century British efforts to produce stronger draft quality in horses to serve urban industry.[21] Neither was distinct from the other. Interbreeding of Clydes and Shires after that time made the Clyde a Scottish version of the same horse, the English Shire.[22] The horses would become redesigned by the end of the nineteenth century because of their involvement with the lucrative transatlantic trade. The hot Duchess Shorthorn craze had not gone unnoticed by livestock people outside the cattle breeds. A deepening interest in the marketing power of purebred breeding became more widespread under these conditions. Clydesdale and Shire breeders reacted to this situation by establishing herd books in order to promote international trade. Breeding habits, however, remained the same. The two types continued to be interbred with each other after the stud book for the Clydesdale was established in Scotland in 1877 and that for the Shire in England in 1878. Initially, when the American Clydesdale Association was formed in 1879, Americans accepted any Clydesdales registered in the British book, and therefore some animals that had Shire crosses.[23]

Within a few years, the promotional activities of two Scottish horse breeders, Lawrence Drew and David Riddell, would lead to profound changes in world of Clydesdale breeding.

In 1883 Drew and Riddell opened a new registry called the Select Clydesdale Horse Society of Scotland. Effectively, they set out to label (not necessarily make) the Clyde as a "breed" and not a "type" while they openly promoted the Clyde/Shire cross in breeding. They claimed legitimacy as to animal background in their stud book registry, but they did not claim purity. Pedigrees in the Select Book were designed to certify quality because they were granted on the basis of "individual merit alone," which would be ascertained by judges at Scottish shows.[24] Selection on the basis of quality and type dominated over selection on the basis of genealogy, as far as Drew and Riddell were concerned. They bred as they had in the past; namely crossing Shires on Clydes.[25] In a lengthy introduction to the new recording book, Drew made it clear how important the Shire had been and still was to quality Clyde breeding. The introduction stated: "The facts which we allege – and we do so without the least hesitation – are these, that ... brood mares alone of the best Clydesdale type which have been brought from England to Scotland within the last forty years [i.e., the English cart horse or Shire] are more than sufficient to account for the ... excellent breed of horses called Clydesdales."[26] Drew also addressed and criticized devotion to the idea of purity. People uneducated in matters of horse breeding, Drew wrote,

> dogmatically assert that the Clydesdale breed of horses is a pure breed, distinct in every sense of the term from the English cart horse, and that it possesses an "impressiveness", whatever that may mean, to which its English neighbour cannot pretend ... What we, on the contrary, assert is that the expressions "Clydesdale horse" and "Shire horse" are synonyms for the same class of animal, and they are no more and no less descriptive of the same type of horse.[27]

The Select Book, by focusing on the issue of quality and not purity, in effect forced Americans to look into the question of how Clydes were actually bred in Scotland. Purity via genealogy had become so central to American views on value in imported stock (animals which they saw as exotic within the North American context) that interest in quality had taken a backseat by this time. Drew and Riddell had underestimated the intense purity-driven climate in the United States when they deliberately designed a registry that openly avoided the revered recording on the basis of genealogy espoused by Americans. Americans did not and would not accept the idea that the Shire was an English version of the Clyde.

In 1886 the American association responded by changing its standards: Shire genetics were no longer permitted in the ancestry of Clydes for registry purposes, and by 1892 the association had managed to get the Scottish Select Society's book off the duty-free list.[28] The downfall of the Scottish Select Society related directly to the American refusal to recognize pedigrees that openly recorded Shire blood. Certification of quality took second place to certification of purity. The rejection of Shire/Clyde breeding by Americans set off a chain of international events. To begin with, Scottish breeders became less likely to have Shires in their Clyde breeding programs, even though the practice of Clyde/Shire crossing continued in a more limited way.[29] In 1895 the secretary of the Clydesdale Horse Society admitted as much when he told a group of breeders at a meeting in Edinburgh that the organization hoped to stop the continuing action of Scottish breeders mating Shire mares with Clyde stallions.[30]

Canada also experienced problems relating to the crossbreeding of Clydesdales, and the Shire/Clyde cross in particular. In the early 1880s, Canadian breeders still routinely imported Clydes from Scotland and crossed these horses on others from various breeds. Their object was more about generating a moderate heavy horse, explicitly for sale to the US, than about purebred breeding (even within the perspective of Clydes with Shire blood). No registry book for Clydesdales or Shires existed in Canada at the time, thereby discouraging widespread concentration on purebred breeding. As one witness reported to the Ontario Agricultural Commission, "my object in crossing the [imported] Clydesdale on Canadian stock is to raise a general purpose horse," one that found a ready market in Toronto, where "Americans come … to buy … all the time, and I think, take them to New York."[31] This horseman apparently believed in breeding heavy, crossbred general horses for the city and industrial market, but specifically for the American market. The international trade in such animals would fall away, however, after 1880, when the American interest in purebred animals mushroomed. While the industrial and city demand for heavy crossbreds remained strong at home, for various reasons Canadian farmers did not find this market particularly attractive (as we saw in chapter 4). Increasingly, however, the emphasis in the United States on purebreds meant greater numbers of them would be imported to Canada and also bred as purebred in Canada.

Canadian importers found it particularly lucrative to focus on the American market. They had a ready outlet for imported Clydesdale horses through exportation to the US. The preponderance of Clydes leaving Britain and destined for North America in these years would, actually, arrive first in Canada, not the United States.[32] Canadians, then, were integral to the new American purebred import story.[33] The Canadian-American linkage in this international trade triggered not only more extensive Canadian pure Clyde breeding but also the establishment of herd books in Canada (the Clyde in 1886 and the Shire in 1888). Clydesdale pedigree standards would subsequently be driven by the American perspective over the years. Canadians set their Clydesdale standards on the basis of the closed system, meaning no input of Shire blood. To provide credibility for horses with Shire/Clyde backgrounds (pedigreed earlier under the four cross system), the Ontario government suggested that Canadian horses of Shire/Clyde cross in future be listed in an appendix.[34] The Clyde breeders favouring the new purity regulations opposed such an action, but the Clyde/Shire story did not end there.

Most Canadians thought the Clyde/Shire cross produced good horses and many believed the crosses were in fact better than pure Clydes or Shires. The issue of pedigrees seemed, however, to be the only thing standing in the way of promoting these good animals. Clyde/Shire producers in Canada decided, therefore, to set up their own, non-appendix-style registry and started to record on the standard basis of accepting Shire blood in Clydes.[35] Since it appeared that a pedigree was all that mattered as far as Americans were concerned, breeders of Clyde/Shire crosses argued that simply pedigreeing the horses in their own separate registry would enable the animals to enter the United States duty free. Apparently they did not understand the implications arising from the difficulties Drew and Riddell had with their Select Clydesdale book, which also maintained accurate pedigrees.

Like Drew and Riddell, Canadian Clyde/Shire producers made every effort to make sure that the records accurately noted the ancestry of the animal. In effect, while these pedigrees showed that the stock was "crossbred," the papers were not bogus. The Drew/Riddell lesson, however, was that Shire/Clyde crosses, even if pedigreed correctly, were unacceptable to Americans. Canadian purebred Clyde breeders, who had rejected even an appendix registry on the basis that Clyde/Shire horses inevitably had no future in the international market, became concerned with these developments. Wanting to protect the redesigned "purebred" Canadian Clyde and Shire in the export business, one such person decided to notify the editor of the *Gazette* about the situation. "We are having trouble here in the draft horse business with new associations, which register and give certificates for cross-bred animals," this Canadian stated, and added "The object is not concealed, viz.: *to give certificates that will help to sell animals on your side*."[36] For the editor of the *Gazette*, this was clearly fraudulent activity, even though the Clyde/Shire breeders were scrupulously careful to make sure that the pedigrees they issued were accurate.

The pedigreeing of so-called crossbreds in Canada made Americans increasingly nervous about purity standards in any imported horses with either Clyde or Shire backgrounds. In 1889 the American Clydesdale Association wanted to impose a registration fee of twenty pounds sterling on all stallions, even recognized purebreds, entering from Canada or Britain. Breeders from these countries were incensed. "As surely as the Clydesdale Association adopts this rule," the *Farmer's Advocate* in Canada said, "as surely will they injure this noble breed and forward the interests of its rivals."[37] Many breeders in Canada continued to support the idea that crossing the Shire on the Clyde provided valuable outcross genetics which brought about hybrid vigour. Such a view, of course, implied that, unlike what Drew claimed about the sameness of the Shire and the Clyde, the two horse types deviated enough (in spite of their similar background breeding over the centuries) to allow for some hybrid vigour from an interbreeding of lines. In 1891 horses registered in the Canadian Clydesdale Association's book (now on the basis of the closed system) had trouble crossing the US border because of confusion over the relationship of the Clyde/Shire stud book to either the Clyde or the Shire books in Canada. Americans found it hard to differentiate these pedigrees from those issued by the Canadian Clydesdale stud book.[38]

As Canadians increasingly came to accept that the American view would direct trade, they were more inclined to refocus on breeding to make it match American market demand. "Our market for draft horses is the United States, and they want pure-bred, not cross-bred, horses, and as long as they want them it is our duty, *as business men*, to breed them," one Canadian wrote in the *Farmer's Advocate*. He continued: "Time and again I see farmers breeding mares with Clyde crosses to Shire stallions, and vice versa, and on remonstrating with them, I am told that they think they will be better horses, and they are breeding horses to suit themselves, not the Americans, and so forth. It makes me tired to hear men talk so; it shows such an utter want of business principles." Farmers can argue all they want that a crossbred horse is better than a purebred one, he said, but when the time comes to sell, they will find that it doesn't pay. Farmers should breed on a business level, not for what they think is the best horse.[39] Breeding, in other words, should always reflect market demand, not quality. Pedigrees were to guarantee and reflect marketability. As with the splintering of traction purpose because of technology, farmers were encouraged to breed for the market, not for what they perceived to be the most useful or the best quality.

Efforts at straightening out the two breeds by recording methods, and the recognition by Americans that pedigrees had been generated for Shire/Clyde animals to make them marketable because of American demands, would sound the death knell for what many believed had been the best type of horse to arise from either the Shire or the Clyde breed: the true Shire/Clyde cross. The resulting Clyde was not the animal that had been bred for so many years before in Scotland. Perhaps it became more consistent as to a type, but it lost the hybrid vigour which knowledgeable breeders could obtain with judicious crossing of Shire mares on Clyde stallions. There is some sense too that the "pure" Clyde lost popularity as a result of its new purity. Certainly other breeds quickly made headway into its North American territory – the Percheron being one, as will be evident below. (The Belgian became a popular horse just before the heavy horse market collapsed forever.)

Pedigrees: Percheron Horses and the Transatlantic Trade, 1880–1910

The French Percheron was another draft type to be forced into the purebred orbit at the same time as the Clyde and Shire. Like them, the Percheron would be redesigned by the conditions of the American import market, but in a somewhat different moulding fashion. In this case, deliberate selection strategies took hold to redesign the phenotype of the Percheron, where in the Clyde/Shire case it was more a question of separating one type from the other. Part of the issue behind the Percheron and its acceptance in the United States was that Americans did not appreciate what the French wanted from their breeding programs. Problems around understanding French breeding emerged as soon as American importation began in 1876, when importers registered the horses in the United States under the name Norman Percheron.[40]

In France, no draft horse was called a Norman, however, and the Percheron type came in several styles, two facts that Americans at first did not recognize. When Americans realized that the word Norman meant nothing to French breeders and that various types of horses qualified as Percherons, they restructured herd books in the United States by dropping the name Norman and then, for import reasons, forced French breeders to breed under the regulations of a registry. Horsemen in the United States, therefore, attempted to change the practices of French breeders by making them adhere both to purebred ideology, which demanded purity of the blood, and to breeding for specific conformation standards.[41] American importers also encouraged French breeders of Percherons to select for greater size and weight in draft horses than the French producers desired. French breeders abandoned the lighter, trotting Percheron type, which they preferred, because of the marketability of the heavier but also awkward and bad-tempered horse that Americans wanted.

French breeders did not always comply with American wishes for change. They, like breeders of cattle in Britain, did not see why it was necessary to pedigree females.[42] The very ubiquity of types made pedigreeing of local animals seem unnecessary, and also made it hard for European breeders to understand that the exotic and rare characteristics of imported animals put them in a completely different category as far as importing countries were concerned. The problem of type and local variation of horses in France continued to puzzle Americans, a situation which encouraged fraudulent activity in both the domestic and import trade. Pedigrees and pedigreeing fed into the situation. Men deliberately brought in poor stock to enhance the comparative appearance of the good animals or to make other breeds compete better with French draft horses. The problem of varying types of French draft horses, and the fluidity of the situation with respect to recording, allowed the deliberate importation of poor quality.[43]

In the late 1880s, the issue of variation in French draft horses and the relationship of types to Percherons finally made the Illinois Board of Agriculture establish a committee to look into the matter of breeds or types in France. Were all French horses in reality Percherons, or did distinct breeds exist in France? The committee concluded that the essence of the problem lay in the fact that pure Percherons were expensive to buy in France, and American importers found that if they could induce men back home to purchase miscellaneous types and breeds from France as purebred Percherons, they made a great deal of money. French authorities were called in and asked what the word "breed" meant in France. These witnesses argued that the word was understood in France to mean the same thing that it did in the United States; namely, distinct types that bred truly.[44] The committee of the Illinois Board came to the conclusion that there were a number of French draft breeds. It was a valuable victory for the Percheron breeders and importers because it undermined a market for other types of French draft horses in the United States which had been claimed to be Percherons. Pedigrees had been the device used to separate types into breeds, and to define what qualities could be found in a distinct breed. French breeders would be forced to work within those guidelines if they wanted to continue exporting to the United States. Notably, attention to actual quality in horse types had played no role in the debate.

Corruption continued, however, in the importing business. "There still remain those," the *Gazette* stated in 1888, "who buy disreputable specimens of horseflesh at merely nominal prices, and with them prey upon the legitimate business of the importer."[45] The problem of fraudulence would cling to the Percheron breed because of this continuing vague definition about the breed of various French horses and the concurrent strong demand for the Percheron itself. The difficulties surrounding French horses would harass farmers in both the United States and Canada as much as, or more than, the Shire/Clyde situation had done. French dealers played a role in that situation. Registered Percheron stallions found to be non-breeders were purchased by dealers from Paris. The dealers wanted the certificate, not the horse, and if they found an American who would buy any particular animal, the certificate would be attached to that horse. It seemed that the same practice was followed in the United States as early as 1887.[46] Pedigrees meant marketing power, a truth unchanged by future conditions.

Pedigrees: Shorthorns and "Invented" Purebred Status in the Transatlantic Trade, 1970–1990

Support for quantitative genetic approaches, which had taken hold in the beef cattle world by the 1970s, had undermined significant purebred breeding principles; most particularly, reverence for ancestry breeding and the consequent emphasis on pedigrees. Unlike the situation in the late nineteenth century, when pedigrees could be more valuable than the cattle, cattlemen appeared ready by this time to put substantial monetary worth on animals regardless of whether or not they qualified for pedigrees. A lucrative demand for various breeds (but types also) resulted from this change in focus and meant that certain grade cattle in Europe, at least by North American standards, could potentially command considerable prices from purebred breeders in the United States and Canada. The story of how Shorthorn importation unfolded as a result of this change of heart, however, shows that newer approaches to pedigrees would have little effect on how the transatlantic trade worked. Attitudes to pedigree standards would not become more relaxed. The cattle had to both acquire pedigrees in the nation of their birth and be accepted via those pedigrees in an importing country if they were to be of any substantial value. Importer and exporter had to make cattle fit into that old pedigree and designated standards mould in order for the trade to take place. In the end, importer and exporter together solved the problem: exporters invented pedigree status for cattle with unknown ancestry backgrounds, and importers subsequently registered those animals on that basis.

The story began with American livestock importer Dick Judy's European search for Simmentals. While in Europe, he took the time to look at cattle from other beef breeds as well. There was a hot market in North America for any type of larger animal in the drive to improve the short blocky stock that the show ring had encouraged in beef cattle over a period of at least fifty years.[47] Judy was aware of that fact when he noticed tall Shorthorn type animals in Ireland, which, as he later learned, did not have pedigrees. The market for large cattle was so hot that he believed he could sell the animals for use on Shorthorns in the United States regardless of lack of recording in Coates's Herd Book. Canadian Shorthorn breeders had also become aware of the Irish animals. Grant Alexander, a Saskatchewan cattleman who was active in the importing business and whose family had been involved with Shorthorns for generations, began buying a year after Judy. He was fully aware of the pedigree status of the cattle but believed they could re-energize North American Shorthorns, through crossbreeding the new arrivals on purebred herds and therefore breeding up to purebred status over four generations.

However, it would be apparent almost immediately that, as far as breeders in North America were concerned, the Irish cattle needed pedigrees in order to be accepted by purebred breeders for breeding purposes.[48] Dick Judy became aware of that fact when the American Shorthorn Association refused to register his new non-registered Irish Shorthorns in their closed book. Discouraged, he started to sell off his devalued imports.[49] Alexander and his partners (under the name Irish Drovers) were prepared to use the new stock for breeding, regardless of its non-pedigreed status in Canada. By breeding up from the non-pedigreed Irish Shorthorns, they argued that fellow Shorthorn breeders could in the end obtain purebred status under the old four cross system. But Canadian breeders would not have it so. They wanted better recognition. When the cattle arrived in Canada, breeders pressed for some sort of registration in the Canadian book. The animals were, as a result, admitted into an appendix (grade or crossbred) Shorthorn book.[50]

Entry into North American herd books would be made easier after Irish exporters began more forcefully to address the problem of pedigrees for their animals purchased by foreign buyers. Irish breeders started eagerly to cooperate with this expanded market by making sure that their animals had pedigrees in Coates's Herd Book. "Many cattle were placed into the herd book if a good bottle of Irish whiskey was involved," Alexander reminisced.[51] Irish breeders often used bulls of unknown background and purchased at local auction marts. Pedigree status had to be manufactured under these conditions.[52] Ancestral background was therefore often invented. The idea of purity, of course, is made nonsense in these international trade patterns. In Alexander's words, "I simply shake my head when I see some of the pedigrees that some people will use in their herd, only because the registration paper says they are pure. Total horse feathers in many cases!!"[53] Because the pedigreeing of Irish cattle eased their entry into North American herd books, a lucrative transatlantic trade exploded. Acceptance in the American book in particular created a market boom. "Once the Irish cattle had registered status in the US, a number of American breeders started making numerous trips to Ireland and the prices of these cattle went through the roof," Alexander noted.[54] The circumstances in Canada changed too. As the international market for Irish cattle mushroomed, Canadians demanded that the cattle be allowed into their closed (purebred) herd book. Alexander and his partners disapproved. "My partners and myself, were totally against this happening," he explained, "as we knew full well that these cattle were appendix at best and more likely truly grades, and I travelled to Vancouver to be able to speak on this motion and try to leave these cattle where they were in the appendix herd book. I was the only opposing vote and it passed."[55]

The events behind this transatlantic cattle trade of the 1970s, which took place long after the decline of government in its affairs, showed that little had changed with respect to the trade's dynamics. The Underwood tariff of 1913 might have ended American government control (through the BAI) of pedigreed stock, but breeder regulations continued to direct the international trade in purebred animals, and did so along historic lines; namely by qualifying what animals were deemed "purebred." If imported animals did not meet the standards of a breeders' national breed registry, the stock could not obtain purebred status and therefore could only come into the importing country devalued as grade or commercial; clearly an impractical state of affairs because of the cost. What makes this transatlantic story especially interesting, however, is that even the quantitative genetic breeding environment of the 1970s for beef cattle could not change historic breeder attitudes to pedigrees and their role in international trade.

Pedigrees: Arabian Horses and the Rise of Global Trade, 1870–2010

The history of the Arabian horse industry adds new dimensions to the story of how pedigree standards shaped the international market by showing, first, that pedigree standards set by breeders and breed associations could shape, not just an international market, but a global one as well; second, animals originally generated outside the purebred method had to be forced into it because of the system's marketing power; and third, significant consequences (for both trade and breeding) would result from the linkage of pedigrees to a particular breeding aim, in this case authenticity (an aim reviewed in chapter 6). Regulatory and monetary ramifications would be huge when pedigree standards reflected a world perspective, when Eastern breeding was viewed through the lens of Western structures, and when authenticity breeding took centre stage.

The animals had been known in Europe long before the beginnings of a global Arabian horse market began, and with it the "Westernizing" of this Eastern type. True "Westernizing" of the Arabian as a breed began in the 1870s, with the importation work of Wilfrid and Lady Anne Blunt at their Crabbet Arabian Stud in England and their concurrent intention not to cross their imports on local stock. The Blunts wanted no breeding up. That approach was new. The Eastern horse had traditionally been used to infuse certain qualities into local horses. The English Thoroughbred, for example, had never been intended, by its cross to these horses, to be "Arabian." The Blunts' desire to establish the Arabian as a Western breed initiated ramifications which would echo throughout the future of the Arabian from a worldwide perspective. To begin with, the horses had to be deemed as purebred. In order for the Arabians imported by the Blunts to be considered a breed or "pure" (and to be marketable as such), they had to have pedigrees on the basis of Western standards. With careful collection of Eastern records, in 1877 the Blunts managed to convince the Weatherby family to allow recording in the General Stud Book (GSB) within a special section.[56] The registration in the GSB of Arabians meant that the horses could be imported from the East and sold to other nations as "purebred," a critical factor when it came to exporting horses. Since the registries of Jockey Clubs in various countries accepted horses with GSB papers, Arabians with a background based on Eastern breeding but also an English pedigree now had easy entry to other European countries as well as the United States.

While an international market trade in Arabians now existed under the regulatory force of GSB pedigrees, other developments with respect to registry systems for Arabians soon came to direct world trade in them. The initiation of a global pedigree-based trade outside the Thoroughbred horse industry began shortly after 1906 in the United States, as a result of actions taken by Homer Davenport, a well-known cartoonist from Oregon. He undertook an importation venture with Arabians which set off a series of events leading to profound changes in how pedigrees related to markets for this Eastern horse. Interested in Arabians with the cavalry in mind, Davenport was convinced that the purest authenticity (and therefore genuine quality) in the horses could be found only in the Arabian's homeland, and therefore he journeyed to the desert looking for horses owned by Bedouin tribes. President Theodore Roosevelt, who also believed that these horses were useful for breeding army horses, provided Davenport with authoritative support, and a wealthy businessman, Peter B. Bradley, funded the endeavour.

Davenport failed to take his twenty-seven imported horses through England and acquire GSB papers before he returned to the United States. As a result, they could not obtain pedigrees in the American Jockey Club's book. In 1906, the Bureau of Animal Industry, which decided what qualified as a purebred animal as a result of the United States Department of Agriculture's role in tariff regulations (set out by the Treasury Department), compelled registration in American books for purebred status. Davenport's Arabians were not eligible for that status, because the only American book that could register Arabians would not accept them. He was forced, therefore, to find another way of pedigreeing his horses. He did so by establishing a new public registry for Arabian horses in 1908, a registry which in time became more dominant than the GSB or the American Jockey Club Book.[57] (The GSB registered Arabians until 1964. Arabians recorded there were acceptable to the American Jockey Club Book up to that time.)

The organization, called the Arabian Horse Club of America, Inc. (renamed several times and finally in 1969 named the Arabian Horse Registry of America, Inc., or AHRA, as it will be referred to here), set up its own rules for recording eligibility. No breeding up would be recognized for purebred status: all horses entered had to be proved to be descended entirely from horses bred in the desert. Davenport's Arabians would have to be grandfathered in, because he had not obtained certificates from the Bedouin breeders giving the horses' ancestry. Any future imported horses, however, would be accepted as purebred by the Arabian Horse Registry of America only if their purity could be authenticated with proper documentation. The mission of the Western registry system was thus to guarantee the Eastern purity of the breed.[58] "It is the purpose and responsibility of the Arabian Horse Registry of America, Inc. to preserve the integrity of the blood of the purebred Arabian horse," read the mission statement of the AHRA.[59] From the beginning, the AHRA defined a pure Arabian as one that came entirely from Bedouin-bred stock, and the organization would pedigree only horses that it believed fitted that description. It was evident as early as Davenport's time that "purity" related to potential marketability. That was his sole reason for founding the new registry. The fact that pedigrees would actually guide how trade operated, however, seemed less clear at the time.

In 1908 the registry accepted Arabian horses from the Jockey Club stud books of Britain, France, Australia, and the United States. Animals recorded in these books qualified for what was called non-discretionary status and were automatically eligible for American pedigrees. Horses not emanating from those sources fell into the discretionary category: they needed supporting documentation to prove their purity, and the directors of the association had the power to accept or reject such documentation. Problems soon emerged over defining what constituted authenticated proof for non-discretionary status, and therefore what purity meant in that context. While the resolution of the registry to preserve purity would not change, what was believed to authenticate such purity would. In 1937, for example, the public stud book of the Polish Arab Horse Breeding Society (founded in 1926) became part of the non-discretionary list, but on the basis of clearly questionable documentation as to purity.[60] The Polish directory often relied on incomplete records of old princely studs. Furthermore, Poles had traditionally bred up from the base of local horses and had never attempted to work with straight Eastern stock. It tended to be directors who owned most Polish horses imported in 1937, a practice which ultimately suggested to some that authenticated purity had simply been a matter of ensuring monetary value and trade potential for the buyers.[61] The assessment of purity in horses outside the non-discretionary books became murkier after 1950. Directors or representatives picked by them had the power to accept or reject horses as to their purity status on a personal and often visual basis.[62]

From the beginning, the American registry found it harder to regulate imports from Eastern countries than from Europe because avenues of entry to the United States from the Middle East made it difficult to evaluate authenticating evidence of pure Bedouin breeding. Over the years, pedigree keeping in the East also shifted in a complex way between private and public recording. The story of the AHRA's attitude to Egyptian Arabians after 1960 illustrates these difficulties. The problem of pedigrees for Egyptian horses arose when the animals came directly from Egypt (not through Europe), from either the government stud (founded in 1914) or private breeding centres. Both types of breeding operations kept pedigrees, but the multiplicity of stud records and the lack of a breeder organization (no association of Arabian horse breeders as a whole existed in Egypt until 1985) made it difficult for the American registry to establish clear-cut qualifications for Egyptian Arabians. The increased American demand for Egyptian Arabians led the AHRA to recognize government-bred Egyptian Arabians in 1964 as a non-discretionary source. The registry also recorded horses from private studs, but in an unclear way as to category – discretionary or non-discretionary. The fact that directors did most of the importing and buying suggested to some people that they deliberately kept the matter imprecise to serve their own interests.[63] Views concerning purity and the authenticity of that purity had, it appeared, to be made to fit pedigree standards. The veracity of documentation concerning the horse's background seemed less important.

The role of pedigrees in world trade and their relationship to the authenticity of the Eastern horse had started to concern Arabian breeders by that time. Apparently how one defined a pure Arabian was intimately connected to a horse's value, and, since definition seemed to vary across countries, no one had a clear understanding of what a pure Arabian was. In 1967 the Arab Horse Society of Britain (which had taken over the recording of Arabians from the GSB) called a meeting of Arabian horse breeders from various nations to discuss forming a world organization for breeders to deal with shared international problems such as purity and its relationship to trade. Representatives from fifteen countries attended, and they created the World Arabian Horse Organization (WAHO). Jay Stream, an American breeder and land developer who grew up on an Iowa farm, was present. He soon became of great importance to the international Arabian horse breeding fraternity.[64] The first job of the new organization was to establish a constitution for it, and at a meeting in London in 1970 Stream agreed to set up a steering committee to develop such a document.

Two years later at the next meeting in Spain, the twenty-seven countries attending ratified the newly designed constitution. WAHO was now able to turn its attention to the problem of international pedigree standards. The organization hoped to streamline the world's stud books into some sort of agreed coordination of the definition of purity.[65] Stream became deeply involved in the problem of international standards and the dichotomies they could present through direct contact with Spanish horses while he was at the 1972 meeting. Stream knew that many of these animals were not acceptable to AHRA, in particular, for registration purposes. The historical background of relatively recent Spanish breeding explains why the AHRA had trouble authenticating the purity of many Spanish horses. The Spanish Civil War had disrupted famous studs – most importantly that of the Duke of Veragua – resulting, not in the loss of the horses, but rather in the loss of pedigrees. Everyone knew the surviving horses were purebred Arabians, but no one could be sure of the correct sires and dams.[66] Important Spanish Arabians recorded in the Spanish national book by the 1960s descended from Veragua mares. Stream managed at least to convince WAHO at the Spanish meeting to accept Spanish horses from Veragua background as purebred and to respect the standards of the Spanish book. Arabians known to have descended from the Duke of Veragua's stud received pedigrees under the name "Veragua."[67] Acceptance by WAHO meant acceptance by the AHRA as a member of WAHO.

The Veragua problem brought the question of conflicting standards directly into the open and also showed how they skewed the market. A new strategy emerged in WAHO out of the controversy on how to deal with clashing standards. If registries in the world could agree on a definition of purebred Arabians, then notions of purity would no longer differ between countries. WAHO members consented to establish a world definition for a purebred Arabian horse, and Stream set out to see that the organization did so. He devoted the next two years to the project. The final definition, accepted in 1974 at the WAHO meeting in Malmö, Sweden, was "a purebred Arabian horse is one which appeared in any purebred Arabian Stud Book or Registry listed by WAHO as acceptable," and the books of thirteen countries were accepted immediately. Members hoped that by 1979 all stud books in the world would be recognized.[68] More stud books did achieve recognition under the WAHO definition of what made an Arabian pure, and by 1986, thirty-seven member countries (which included the AHRA) had their record books approved.[69] "The biggest contribution that WAHO has made is to standardize the stud books to some extent and to require enough recording on import-exports so that we know in fact that the horse actually coming into the country matches his papers," remarked Stream.[70] Central to this question of accepting such a definition of purity would be the position taken on it by the AHRA. Because the AHRA controlled what horses could enter the United States as purebred, and because American trade also drove the international market, registries in countries where the AHRA would not recognize pedigrees could not command the respect of the Arabian horse community of the world. Under these conditions, quality did not dictate acceptance in the United States or ultimately in that wider community. The AHRA was a member of WAHO, but would it abide by pedigree decisions put forward by WAHO?

By the 1980s the Arabian Horse Registry of America, as a member of WAHO from the beginning, began telling the world organization that, although it intended to accept WAHO's definition of purity, it needed time to do so. At the same time, the AHRA rejected all pedigrees from 35 per cent of WAHO countries, even though delegates from the AHRA had voted in favour of all the policies these countries followed.[71] The AHRA stood by its claim that it protected the purity of the breed. The organization would not, in effect, even address the idea that it might always have seen the issue of purity and its authenticity as a way of manipulating pedigrees in order to direct trade and guide monetary value. The purity issue (in the context of pedigree recognition and documented evidence of purity) came to a head over descendants of the German stallion Kurdo III, imported in 1910 to Argentina, where he produced many offspring. Although accepted by WAHO, his pedigree indicated that he might have descended from a Thoroughbred mare, 30 Maria, born in 1842 and registered in the GSB.[72] In the 1990s the AHRA rejected the WAHO decision by refusing to recognize the pedigrees of certain Argentinean horses that had descended from the controversial stallion. WAHO reacted to this situation by agreeing at its 1996 meeting in Abu Dhabi to suspend the AHRA in February 1997 unless it agreed to accept WAHO's definition of a purebred Arabian, and therefore all horses recognized by WAHO as pure Arabians. The AHRA justified its actions by claiming that, by rejecting Kurdo III, it protected the purity of the breed.

The international market for Arabians broke down under these conditions. While many Arabians would be barred from entry into the United States, WAHO countries, in turn, would no longer accept American-registered horses for import into their nations. Some members of WAHO believed that it made no sense to ostracize the largest single registry in the world, or to threaten the world's largest market for Arabians.[73] The AHRA did not take long to feel the isolation and in 1998 signed a bilateral agreement with Jordan for trade in purebred stock between the two countries.[74] The AHRA began to look for other allies, and by late 2001 had succeeded in establishing a new Arabian horse breeding union. The registry completed negotiations with countries in the Americas – most of them also members of WAHO – to create an organization called the Alliance of the Americas, which represented 75 per cent of the world's Arabians.

When it abandoned a policy of isolation, however, the AHRA re-entered the world of international pedigrees and the problem of relating them to each other. Nothing had changed. The AHRA found, for example, that it was forced to alter its earlier position on an issue that had precipitated the break with WAHO. The registry agreed to grant pedigree status to certain South American horses previously designated by the association as impure for recording purposes.[75] The AHRA's *volte face* over the South American horses provided clear evidence that its arguments concerning the meaning of purity were dichotomous. The underlying power of pedigrees to direct trade and create value, not the belief that standards related to purity, drove the way the AHRA's pedigreeing system for international horses evolved. The organization had difficulty making the existence of faulty pedigrees fit with its mission statement to preserve purity because of that basic concern with markets. By 2001 it was entirely evident to members of the AHRA (pointed out repeatedly as well by WAHO) that the American registry itself was not free of impure pedigreed horses, a situation which undermined its credibility in relation to its mission statement. The weakened and obviously dichotomous (and often self-serving) position of the AHRA concerning purity ultimately led to its demise: in 2003 it merged with a second American association to form the Arabian Horse Association (AHA). By 2007 the AHA had become a member of WAHO.

The WAHO versus AHRA debate shows that even when concerted efforts were made to straighten out conflicting standards in order to ease trade and to make sense of faulty recording in pedigrees, contentious issues remained in place. The persistent view that pedigrees proved purity and quality does much to explain why it was so difficult to solve these trade problems. Pedigree standards from the time they were used to direct trade after 1880 have continued to be critical to international trade in Arabians. Adherence to WAHO standards remained critical. Any country whose registry was rejected by WAHO would in turn be rejected by the registries of WAHO members.

Purity by Western standards became, therefore, just as important in Egypt as elsewhere. It had to be preserved in order to take part in the global market which had evolved by 1980. Even Arab people in Kuwait, Morocco, Saudi Arabia, and Qatar bought Egyptian Arabians bred in Europe and the United States as well as in Egypt itself by the 1980s, and continued to do so into the 1990s and beyond.[76] Much of the enthusiasm for these horses rested on the conviction that the animals represented maintenance of past glories derived from ancient Bedouin breeding.[77] Egyptian Arabians would be seen as a national and ethnic symbol of Arab culture by Arab breeders, thereby feeding heavily into the new global sense of authenticity. Under this impetus, the implications of breeding for authenticity reached new heights from a trade perspective. Market forces in conjunction with the ethos of authenticity played an increasingly important role in the breeding success of Egyptian Arabian horses. The animals supported a global vision, but they also drove a global market.

It behooved any country to make sure that all its national pedigrees met WAHO standards, even if that meant exclusion of certain lines whose claim to purity and authenticity were beyond question. That situation would raise a problem in Egypt for certain breeders. The Egyptian breeder registry barred certain lines of recognized Arabians in that country because their records could not conform to WAHO standards. The registry refused national recognition of the Tahawi Arabians, which everyone knew had been generated by Bedouin Tahawi people (living in Egypt since the time of Mohammed Ali) from pure imported Bedouin stock. The horses were ineligible for pedigrees under the national registry because of their lack of Western-style accurate records, a situation which resulted at least partially from the fact that the breeders of this type of stock tended to rely on Bedouin practices of testing their horses for ability rather than beauty and pedigree for breeding purposes. Tahawi Arabians had been valued by the royal studs of the nineteenth century, but under present conditions, set in accordance with WAHO, they have become devalued.[78] It might be claimed that Egyptian horses represent authenticity of pure Bedouin breeding, but the rigid adherence to Western purebred standards (far stronger than in the early days of the government breeding programs and at the height of importation to the US in the 1960s) makes that claim questionable in light of the reality that the linkage of such breeding to markets is undeniable.

~

Pedigrees played a vital role in all stories about the livestock trade. Even early in the nineteenth century, pedigrees proved how valuable they could be in international trade, as the Shorthorns imported by Renick show in relation to the Seventeens. Pedigrees as such could be traded as valuable commodities, and the Duchess boom of the 1870s was a climax of that phenomenon. That pedigrees could also be used as instruments to promote trade by shaping breeds can be seen in the invention of registries between 1980 and 2000 for two crossbred types of horses under Gene LaCroix Jr, thereby creating new breeds. Fraudulent pedigree activity in the late nineteenth century triggered the movement for stallion legislation, and a review of opinions held about the issue offers a particularly rich impression of what the average horseman thought about heredity, the relationship of purebred standards to good breeding, and their work in contrast to that of elites.

Canadian-American trade patterns made clear as early as 1880 that making Canadian standards conform to American ones was vital to cross-border trade. Acceptance of pedigrees by Americans would be just as important to the transatlantic purebred trade between the exporting countries and North America as it had been in the Canada-US situation.[79] The use of pedigrees as tariffs, on top of the general move to the idea that purity defined quality, could even bring about the demise of breeding practices known to produce good stock. The declining welfare of Clyde/Shire cross horses in North America and the shift to a different phenotypic style in Percherons indicated how significant pedigrees as tariffs, combined with notions of purity in pure breeds, could be to breeding techniques and to the development of breeds from what had been types. Pedigrees could be so important to the transatlantic trade in cattle that sometimes they had to be invented. Such was the case when breeders brought Irish Shorthorn types to North America for breeding up purposes. Importers had not been interested in purity or even purebred status in such animals. The stock was wanted for breeding up local Shorthorns in order to increase the size of the animals, but recording was so critical to these plans that both exporters and importers found they needed the invention of pedigrees for the Irish cattle.

The WAHO versus AHRA debate emanated from pedigree standards issues. The Arabian horse industry, at the turn of the twenty-first century, showed patterns that had been prevalent since the 1880s when it came to trade guided by pedigrees. These patterns, though, apparently had global implications when it came to international trade. The WAHO story demonstrated that attempts at world organization to overcome the problem of clashing national standards did not necessarily make the market work more effectively, nor could global association define what either quality or purity meant. Pedigrees still count (as do their standards) and still direct market value.

Final Remarks

Animal breeding patterns as we know them today began to evolve at the end of the eighteenth century in Western Europe with the rise of improvement breeding and the decline of environmental breeding. Animal breeding methods would develop from the intent to improve under adherence to the force theory, which postulated that no understanding of hereditary laws was necessary in order to develop a workable breeding methodology. An innate affinity of naturalist or geneticist with practical breeders developed over time from a mutual allegiance to force theory as the fundamental way to view the process of heredity. From the beginning, the practical animal breeding world could interface, either simultaneously or as a result of exchange, with the thinking of force theory naturalists. The situation around pedigree keeping as an avenue to explain heredity serves as an example. Selection under purebred breeding rested on complex views about ancestry and consistency but relied on pedigrees (or some sort of chart) to measure degrees found in individual animals. This practical "law" reflected a breeder interpretation of how the hereditary force functioned, as was clearly laid out by the master American chicken breeder I.K. Felch as early as 1877. The similarity to Francis Galton's late nineteenth-century force theory approach, via his Ancestral Law, is stunning.

When sections of Western naturalist and later scientific thinking about improvement breeding shifted away from that force theory, the animal breeding situation became increasingly complicated. The rise of cell or gene architecture theory, which argued that the dynamics and nature of the force had to be understood before any proper breeding could proceed, lay at the bottom of new conflicts and subsequent divisions. There were indications that practical breeders at least took notice of the new cell (or gene architecture) approach to animal breeding, even if they were not overtly influenced by it. H.H. Stoddard, an American chicken breeder, would be fascinated by Mendelism and wondered if in the future it could be useful for practical animal breeding. Theoretically, Mendelism undermined the conviction that pedigrees could be used to explain laws of heredity, as British Collie breeder William Mason recognized shortly after 1900. Apparently, inheritance of recessive characteristics denied the consistency in animals that pedigrees implied, Mason explained to fellow Collie dog breeders. Recessive or poor characteristics could reappear in future generations regardless of attempts to breed them out by selection based on an animal's background.

Those adhering to genetic architecture theory tended by the late twentieth century to see the force theory in terms of black box thinking, implying an acceptance of ignorance. Developments in molecular biology after 1970, particularly the technology of recombinant DNA, enhanced that sense. But the practical breeder outlook, even if it was a black box approach, had over the centuries led to industry implications outside breeding methodology, and these in the end did much to explain the fate of gene architecture methodology. When the historic structure of animal breeding industries is taken into account, it is evident that the theoretical cleavage between force and gene architecture attitudes did much to explain what supported the infiltration of science into practical breeding, and also factors behind why that was the case. Methodology emanating out of force theory (particularly Bakewellianism and purebred breeding) had historically developed in tandem with industry structure, which was based on a firm linkage between breeder and producer. Force theory methods worked seamlessly with the breeder-producer linkage because of its emphasis on true line breeding. For genetic architecture theory methods to function in a breeding industry, the linkage, and therefore industry structure as well, had to be broken. In other words, a naturalist (or geneticist) adherence to force theory lent itself to the practical breeding world, because no deviation from basic industry structure was implied. The success of gene architecture (or hybridist) methodology in animal breeding would largely be governed by how weak the breeder-producer linkage was.

The cattle breeding industry serves as an example of how future cooperation between geneticist and practical breeder would work under force theory. The 1940s to 1970s interface between genetics and practical animal breeding within the cattle industries was successful because, first, the two groups worked from the foundation that no genetic laws need be understood in order to breed properly. Both, in effect, supported a black box premise. Second, the linkage of breeder to producer was not threatened. The move by breeders to supporting quantitative genetics interfaced well with the historic structure of the industries which developed over a two-hundred-year period to orchestrate the production of true breeding lines. Quantitative genetics, then, fitted with practical breeding theory, methodological intent, and industry structure. While the analogy of black box theory became attached specifically to quantitative genetics, in the end it could also be used to describe classic genomic approaches to animal breeding methodology. There are signs that developments in epigenetics could follow the same course.

Selective breeding for improvement under classic force theory methodology would be driven by many aims, all of which played a significant part in the culture and philosophic foundations of various animal breeding industries. Sometimes breeding aims seemed at odds with the primary focus of modern breeding. The drive to manipulate animals, so basic to nineteenth- and twentieth-century purebred breeding, could, for example, be seen as leading to a lack of improvement (or, even worse, degeneration) when it resulted in pronounced phenotypic change in animals. Even the fundamental idea of heredity as a force came under attack when this point of view was held. In these conditions, facets of environmental breeding took centre stage, indicating that apparently support for the pre-eighteenth-century views on heredity had not completely died in the West. Animal type was considered to be best when it remained true to what was perceived to be its original version, which would have emerged under environment breeding systems. The ideology behind authenticity breeding rests on the premise that adherence to original phenotype should guide selection strategies. This devotion to authenticity as a valid breeding aim suggests that a vision, almost crusade-like in nature, could play an important role in what breeding practices would be followed. Clearly philosophic and cultural concerns could drive breeding decisions.

When Western breeding culture came to adhere to the principles of purebred breeding in the latter half of the nineteenth century, reliance on pedigrees to orchestrate trade quickly took centre stage. By the late nineteenth century, organizations that supported purebred breeding decided how pedigrees would operate by setting standards for entry into the registry. In the process they came to act as the executive head of the breeding procedure. These bodies not only launched pedigree registries which publicly detailed the genealogical background of animals belonging to a breed but also established standards for entry into that registry. The breed associations, in effect, regulated what animals could be described as "purebred." Standards were originally designed to show and guarantee innate quality in the stock so that other breeders could make breeding decisions on the basis of an animal's background.

That idea quickly became superseded by the importance of trade that pedigrees conferred. Pedigrees would be devices to guide how trade would operate. As instruments with market implications, they swiftly showed more wide-ranging consequences. Designed to control the process of heredity, pedigrees instead played havoc with many trade aspects of animal breeding industries.

The history of trade in Arabian horses provides a significant illustration of the upheaval that pedigree standards and their regulation of markets, in conjunction with tensions between improvement breeding aims and environmental or authenticity breeding aims, could trigger. When Western horsemen began to focus on the Eastern Arabian, more complex issues around pedigrees, recording standards, and the historical implications of improvement and environmental breeding came to the fore. Western breeders revered authenticity in the Arabian's Eastern breeding and set out to preserve trueness to that historic type. The North American meshing of Western and Eastern methods, as well as a combined improvement and environmental stance towards breeding, initiated a move to globalize breeding aims in relation to the Arabian horse on a world scale. Shifting Eastern views would cement that process.

Western demand for Eastern animals might have initiated a slow process of incorporating the Eastern ethos with the Western, but at the same time Eastern breeders were affected. At first they found themselves confronted with an ideology somewhat foreign to them. They would, however, absorb certain Westernized attitudes. By the end of the twentieth century, Eastern breeders had adopted both Western strategies and pedigreeing standards, while maintaining some of their ancient culture, which also rested on the dream of authenticity to historic type. The result was what might be called a new, transnational or global approach to breeding methodology, culture, and regulation. The story of the Arabian horse in the East and the West over centuries suggests explanations for many dichotomous aspects found throughout the modern world of breeding. It seems likely that authenticity has played a role in conflicting views that have become increasingly prevalent in other national, international, and global animal industries.

It is interesting to focus on the purity issue within the framework of the three main themes of this book. Purity has been of considerable concern to historians who study the culture of animal breeding, as well as its relationship to eugenics. That situation makes it particularly worthwhile to assess it within the shape of *Made to Order*. It becomes obvious, when purity is positioned as a matter of breeding method, breeding aim, and trade, that there is no straightforward and linear explanation for why it was so important to animal breeding. It is too simplistic, for example, to argue that the purity vision was just a transposition of eugenic thinking from people to animals, or, vice versa, that purity in animals served primarily as a justification for concerted efforts to follow eugenicist improvement plans directed at the human race.

The idea of purity in animals originated with Thomas Bates's system of purebred breeding between 1835 and 1850. Bates masterfully structured his purity vision so that it had three different, valuable, and even separate thrusts which fitted neatly into the three themes of this book. Any one of these could take centre stage at some point in the history of animal breeding. Of primary importance (and arguably most essential in the long run, because it underpinned all other purity aspects) was Bates's vision of purity as a breeding method (section one), one which he saw as a way to achieve consistency in animals. Purity, in effect, could even be used to define the meaning of breed, because the idea of "breed" rests on consistency of type. Basic in early times to I.K. Felch's breeding system, and in keeping with Galton's Ancestral Law, breeding for purity as a way to maintain consistency has continued to dominate many animal industries (regardless of Mendelism's theory of recessive inheritance). In relation to section two, Bates's vision of purity became a primary breeding aim with various ramifications. Tesio, the Italian Thoroughbred horse breeder, saw the purity aim in breeding as one promoting energy or power in horses, and therefore the drive to win. Purity as lack of contamination would be fundamental to the authenticity breeding aim. It could in reality, however, be hard to differentiate, or distinguish, purity as a breeding aim from authenticity as a breeding aim. Arabian horse breeders' adherence to Bedouin strain theory, for example, might have been a purity breeding aim designed to avoid contamination, but it might also have been solely driven by an effort to maintain authenticity. It was in a purity linkage to trade or monetary concerns (section three), however, that we perhaps see Bates's greatest achievement. By associating either a purity breeding method or a purity breeding aim with this third factor, namely the market, Bates created a powerful system which rested on an interconnected and linked triangle. Examples of how that purity-based triangle operated are endless. It explained the growth of the transatlantic trade for cattle and horses in the late nineteenth century, the rise of a global market for Arabian horses over the twentieth century, the fate of the Hereford bull Perfection's descendants, and the acceptance of Irish Shorthorns after 1970.

It is true that Burke's Peerage had been published by the time Bates's triple vision of purity arose, and also that Bates likely knew of the public's interest in aristocratic genealogy (or what might be termed the breeding of the nobility). The fact that he capitalized on purity as a three-pronged feature of animal breeding, however, suggests to me that animal purity cannot be simply extrapolated to mean that animal breeding equals human aristocratic breeding. Animal purity was clearly far more complicated than this simple equation would suggest. By addressing purity in the framework of this book, one can see how its impact affected the dynamics of animal breeding and why that impact could be both so complicated and so powerful.

This book's overview approach to the subject of breeding and its impact over the years reveals and also explains other complex patterns evident in livestock production today. It is unmistakable, for example, how important (and pervasive) the trend to breeding quantitatively over generations for true breeding lines has been when it comes to the manipulation of animals. Hybridizing for terminal crosses is critical to present-day chicken breeding and has played a significant historical and modern role in pig breeding. Both such breeding strategies, however, rely on true breeding lines, synthetic or otherwise. These are the tools for hybrid breeding, and as such they remain important for hybrid breeding industries. It is important to note, however, that synthetic lines owned and developed by breeding companies are never for sale. Such lines serve as tools for the corporate bodies that invented them in order to produce the stock the companies sell – animals for use and not for breeding.

When it comes to a discussion about the trade in breeding material, it is not possible to talk about the lines developed by the chicken or pig breeding companies. The only way to obtain the genetic base leading to terminal hybrid results is to steal it. As one geneticist remarked recently, the corporate breeding industry is "an industry of thieves."[1] The fact that corporate breeding material is never on the market means that true breeding lines in this case are truncated. The practices and culture of creating animals that breed truly and play a role in the marketplace comprise a different story and one which dominates this book. *Made to Order* shows how breeding both evolved and subsequently led to the circulation of animals as well as the ideas behind what created them, within the framework of hereditary theory, method of breeding, reasons or breeding aims, and markets. When people generally are able to acquire and work with the basic material of true breeding lines, artificial selection takes on many interesting features, resulting in constant change within animal populations. The vast panorama of human thought, society, evolving knowledge, and use of animals becomes evident.

There also appears to be a widespread sense in humans that animals should be bred to consistent and standardized styles, in whatever fashion that is done. Standardization ideology lay behind much of that need to develop registry systems, breed standards, and exhibition structures. All supported trade in a standardized commodity. The history of the purebred dog industry serves as a case in point. Purebred, standardized dogs might have seen reduced popularity, but it is important to note that the newer so-called crossbred types are in fact really new synthetic breeds. They may be composites of different breeds, but they have become regulated and standardized in much the same fashion.

Purebred breeding as a force is very much with us, in spite of new ideas about what a "breed" is, erosion of some of its principles, and, even more important, innovations arising from both genetics and technology. The purebred system seems to have developed a new role: namely to orchestrate how innovative trends could mesh with older ways. While quantitative genetics played a major role in the breeding of purebred cattle by the 1970s (as would genomics after 2010), its incursion resulted in remnants of purebred breeding remaining in place. Genomic profiling and DNA defect testing also became incorporated with purebred breeding. How to fully characterize modern purebred breeding or explain why, in its own right, it still seems so authoritative, however, remains difficult. Perhaps we should be looking more at how purebred breeding functioned historically in the development of livestock industry structures and the organization of market systems, and then at how breeding proceeded under purebred standards. Clearly it is the purebred system's organization of pedigreeing, above all its other aspects, that has remained essential to the livestock industries. In essence, it would appear, purebred breeding has adjusted to the infiltration of quantitative genetics and the decline of purity as a breeding value by maintaining power over the regulation and orchestration of trade in animals.

Perhaps a good way to end this book is to elaborate on how the three themes dealt with in *Made to Order* can explain puzzling dichotomies. Section one on theory in relation to methodology indicates that the rise of improvement breeding introduced significant new attitudes. Animals, I would argue, became more "other" than had been the case under environmental breeding, when selection was a haphazard affair relating to environmental conditions. After that time animals would increasingly become appreciated as objects to be used and manipulated, a situation which went hand in hand with a growing emphasis on animals as marketable commodities. By the late nineteenth century and throughout the twentieth, the linkage of monetary worth with the breeding of animals had become so dominant that it concealed the fact that other issues influenced how breeders operated. It is here that section two on specialization is particularly valuable. Through an assessment of specialization it begins to become evident that hidden factors, masked by the prominence of monetary concerns, had always been part of breeding. The desire for authenticity, for example, was driven with different ends in mind, and had both ethical and aesthetic undertones. On the other hand, specialization for what appears clearly to be based on fancy – breeding for colour, for example – might reflect an interest in breeding for sport, or complicated marketing issues arising from the structure of the livestock industry. The move to breeding for a single purpose, while encouraged by economic considerations, revealed other interesting undercurrents which separated money from breeding, and even separated men from women, philosophically speaking. In some ways the feminine attitude harked back to that more commonly seen under environmental breeding. Section three, pedigrees and regulations, emphasizes the importance of pedigrees to all aspects of trade. Any outside observer, appreciating how significant the trade and pedigree connection was but failing to look at it in light of other factors, would get the wrong impression: namely, that breeders were activated simply to make money.

Animal breeding is an ancient human practice, and there is little to say it won't continue to be important in the future, or that historic patterns in it will change. Its past and present tell us much about how human thinking, theorizing, and evolving approaches characterize our interaction with all natural processes.

Glossary

AHRA Arabian Horse Registry of America, a registry for American Arabians.

ancestral law Founded by Francis Galton in 1897. The law states that heredity input to an individual is based on percentage input of ancestors by generation. Parents would each be half and grandparents each a quarter, for example. It is a matter of percentages in relation to generations. The law does not take into account dominant or recessive inheritance characteristics.

ancestry breeding Selecting animals for breeding on the basis of their parents or more remote ancestors.

authenticity breeding Selecting animals for breeding on the basis of trueness to historic type.

Bakewellian breeding principles Breeding via inbreeding and selection on the basis of the progeny test.

bioinformatics and functional genomics The study of the dynamics of the DNA molecule in its entirety, that is the functioning of so-called junk DNA with regions of DNA that code for protein (areas known to influence how characteristics are inherited). (See SNPs; gene.)

biological lock Breeding that results in progeny that will not replicate themselves, compelling the buyer to go back to the breeder for the next generation.

biometry The statistical study of inheritance of variable traits within populations. A form of classical genetics. (See traits as quantitative.) Founded by Francis Galton.

black box theory or thinking When certain results can be attributed to causes, but the laws governing those causes are unknown.

BLUP (best linear unbiased prediction) A statistical model designed to predict an animal's breeding potential under environmentally neutral conditions. (See sire indexing.)

breeding up The crossing of a purebred animal on local grade stock over four generations in order to "breed up" to purebred status. It would be a matter of percentage.

cell theory The argument that inheritance is controlled by knowable physical or cell matter.

Charolais A French beef cattle breed.

chromosome A stretch of DNA containing many genes and other nucleotide sequences. Species have different numbers of chromosomes. Sex chromosomes govern the sex of the offspring and other characteristics that are linked with sex inheritance. Autosome chromosomes carry the rest of genetic hereditary information.

closed herd book A registry which pedigrees animals only if the sire and dam are also pedigreed. (See four cross system.)

cow/calf operators Farmers who keep cows and breed them for calves to be raised for beef. Cow/calf operators act as multipliers but also breeders through choices they make when breeding their cows to certain bulls.

CRISPR Cas 9 A technology capable of manipulating, and therefore altering, the structure of the genome's DNA.

crossbred Animals that result from the crossing of two distinct breeds.

crossbreeding The mating of animals not related to each other. They can belong to the same breed or different breeds.

dosage theory A statistical way to breed Thoroughbred horses on the basis of ancestry percentage charts.

double cross hybrid breeding method The inbreeding of four separate lines, and subsequent crossing of these inbred lines to produce two new inbred lines based on the original four. A final cross comes from breeding the two new inbred lines to each other.

double helix Describes the shape of DNA molecules, in which two long chains of nucleotide subunits twist around each other, forming a right-handed helix. There are four bases in the chains – A (adenine), T (thymine), G (guanine), or C (cytosine). They join each other in the following manner: where one strand has an A, the other has a T, and where one has a G, the other has a C. Species differ only by the sequence of the A, G, T, and C nucleotides. (See SNPs.)

ENCODE The mapping of critical repeat sections of DNA.

epigenetics The term, invented as early as 1949, for the theory that unknown forces (such as environmental) outside the functioning of DNA affect inheritance.

environmental breeding The breeding of animals on the basis of controlling environmental factors, usually in order to maintain quality and prevent deterioration.

EPD (estimated progeny difference) An EPD is a prediction of an animal's likelihood of passing on a trait in relation to breed average for that trait.

evolutionary synthesis The union of various aspects of biology. The synthesis, which developed over the 1930s, reunited ideas emerging from various facets of the general discipline (such as genetics, cytology, systematics, ecology, and palaeontology), and in the process explained how natural selection, that is Darwinian evolution, worked. As far as the science of genetics was concerned, the evolutionary synthesis made Mendelism compatible with biometric principles, and in doing so provided for the rise of population and quantitative genetics.

feeders, or feeder farmers A group of farmers who specialize in feeding out beef cattle for slaughter.

figure system The breeding of Thoroughbred horses on the basis of ancestral root mares in an animal's pedigree.

force theory The idea that an unknown matter in an animal acted as a force to govern how inheritance worked. Force theory argued that a general force comprising innate but unknown biological material, not the environment, directed what the progeny from breeding would be like. The workings of the general force could be assessed by the outcome of any breeding strategy, making it unnecessary to know what constituted the force or how it worked.

four cross system Breeding up to purebred standard over four generations.

gene (or genetic) A stretch of DNA that codes for protein, meaning that it specifies how the protein used to build cells in the body will develop and function.

gene (or genetic) architecture approach A way of understanding the process of heredity, based on the concept that the functioning of genes had to be understood before a successful breeding method could be developed. (See cell theory. Opposed to force theory breeding.)

genomics The study of DNA at the molecular level but across all chromosomes in any given species. A form of molecular genetics.

genotype The genetic makeup of an individual. Not observable by assessing the physical animal.

GSB General Stud Book, the British registry for the Thoroughbred horse.

heifer A young female cow that has not yet calved.

heterosis An explanation for hybrid vigour, which is based on the theory that a return to heterozygosis from homozygosis brings about increased vigour. (See heterozygosis; homozygosis.)

heterozygosis If an animal inherits a trait in a dominant/recessive way, it is heterozygotic to that trait, meaning that while it might itself demonstrate one form of the trait, it can transmit another. Such an animal will not breed truly for a certain form of that trait. (See crossbreeding.)

homozygosis A uniform inheritance of traits, on either a double dominant or double recessive basis. If an animal is homozygotic for a trait, it can pass only one form of that trait to its offspring. It will, therefore, breed truly in connection with that trait. (See inbreeding.)

hybrid animals or plants Usually, stock produced by hybridizing, meaning the creation of two inbred lines and the subsequent crossing of those lines.

hybrid vigour Found in progeny who are superior to their parents because of crossbreeding or hybridizing. Hybridizing is a method of breeding which relies on the crossing of two separate inbred lines. Hybrid vigour occurs only in the first-generation cross.

hybridizing or hybrid breeding The breeding of two individuals in an effort to gain hybrid vigour or superiority in the offspring. The offspring, however, will not breed truly to their improvement. Hybrid breeding can be done across breeds, across inbred lines within a breed, or across species. Hybridizing is commonly associated with the method that calls for the inbreeding of two separate lines and the subsequent crossing of those lines. (See heterosis.)

improvement breeding Manipulation of animals by breeding strategies. It replaced environmental breeding (namely the preservation of type) in the West.

inbreeding The mating of animals closely related to each other. In and in breeding means intense inbreeding.

individual worth Selecting individual animals for breeding on the basis of their performance.

infinitesimal model of inheritance A theory that explains how quantitative traits are inherited. It states that traits are regulated by a large number of segregating Mendelian units acting together.

LD (linkage disequilibrium) The non-random association of nucleotides at two or more loci, meaning that more variation (polymorphism) in genetic markers (at loci) occurs in a population than would be expected in random formation. (See SNPs.)

mass selection Selecting animals for breeding from a group on the basis of certain characteristics. The favouring of various individuals according to some set criteria (such as looks or production history).

Mendelism The study of heredity on the basis of Mendel's laws. A form of classical genetics.

microsatellites Repeating sequences of base pairs in DNA. They can be used as genetic markers to explain the presence of certain characteristics.

molecular genetics The study of inheritance at the DNA level; the study, therefore, of genetic architecture.

naturalists People who questioned all aspects of nature and theorized on laws driving any known phenomenon. A word used to describe what would become, after 1900, scientists. In the terms of this book, naturalists were eighteenth- and nineteenth-century versions of twentieth-century geneticists.

open herd book A registry that pedigrees animals if their purity to the breed has reached a certain level. Normally that situation results from breeding up over generations from a base grade to what is then defined as a purebred.

outcrossing Effectively the same as crossbreeding. The breeding of unrelated lines, meaning crossing breeds or crossing inbred lines.

path coefficient A way of calculating the level of shared genetic material that would result from different inbreeding systems – brother to sister, first cousins, double first cousins, half-brother to half-sister, and so on. An accurate quantitative way to measure the level of homozygosis resulting from any type of inbreeding.

phenotype Observable characteristics in an animal; its physical appearance.

population genetics The study of inheritance of qualitative traits within the framework of populations. A form of classical genetics. (See traits as qualitative.)

postgenomics The period, roughly after 2010, following the mapping of DNA genomes.

progeny testing Selection of animals for breeding purposes on the basis of their progeny.

purebred breeding Selection of individuals for breeding on the basis that both have registered pedigrees in a public herd book.

pure lines Animals that breed truly to type over generations. Normally associated with the idea of breed.

quantitative genetics The study of the inheritance of quantitative traits in populations. A form of classical genetics. (See traits as quantitative.)

QTL (quantitative trait loci) The loci of genetic material proven to relate to productive traits in livestock. The loci can be genes, or even simply stretches of DNA that do not code for protein (meaning they do not specify how the protein used to build cells in the body will develop and function) if these stretches are known to be close to the genes that regulate traits sought after.

recombinant DNA The transferring of sections of DNA from one organism into another, in order to study and manipulate that DNA. Recombinant DNA technology opened the possibility of studying genetics at the DNA level, and laid the basis for genomics.

Simmental A breed of beef cattle from France, Germany, and Switzerland.

sire indexing A sire index for dairy bulls works on the assumption that the level of inheritance of a daughter's ability to produce milk is halfway between that of her sire and her dam, and that by knowing the milk-producing level of dam and daughter, one can calculate the sire's transmitting ability. With no daughters yet in existence, a young male's breeding potential value can only be calculated on the basis of an average value between that of his two parents, namely his mother's milking ability and his sire's ability to produce good daughters.

SNPs (single nucleotide polymorphisms) An evident deviation in an individual or group from population-norm sequencing patterns of the four bases in the DNA molecule. The insertion or deletion of an AT or GC unit, making that variation. (See double helix.)

standardbred breeding The selection of animals for breeding on the basis of meeting a recognized standard.

synthetic lines A group of animals that reproduce truly but were created by systems of inbreeding and crossing inbred lines. Not seen as a breed, but in many ways similar to a breed.

Thoroughbred breeding The name applied only to the breeding of the Thoroughbred horse, which originated from the crossing of Arabians on local British horses, thereby making the animals "thoroughly" bred. Critical to Thoroughbred breeding was the public stud book.

training population A group of animals whose profiles are used to establish a template for superior DNA profiles.

traits as qualitative Traits that separate one species from another. With the advent of the science of genetics, early Mendelists believed that all differences were fundamentally qualitative, meaning they were not explained by inheritance factors and therefore were discontinuous from generation to generation. Today when traits are looked at qualitatively, they are studied under population genetic theory, which addresses evolution. Traits only become qualitative when it can be said that they divide one species from another.

traits as quantitative The view that variation and differences in traits occur because they are inherited in a quantitative way, that is on the basis of amount – more or less. The biometricians, in opposition to the Mendelists, believed all inherited differences were primarily quantitative and therefore continuous from generation to generation. Today when traits are studied quantitatively, the focus is on changes over short generational spans (such as better meat production and milk yields in cattle, or egg laying in chickens), and not on evolution. Traits in farm animals are looked at quantitatively under quantitative genetic theory, in order to find better ways to predict the outcome of breeding strategies.

transgenics The trans-positioning of certain genetic material from one organism into another.

true breeding The breeding of animals that will largely replicate themselves in the next generation.

unit character theory The theory that quantitative traits are inherited on the basis of a single gene.

WAHO The World Arabian Horse Organization, a body which directs standards for pedigree on a global scale in relation to Arabian horses.

Warmbloods Horse breeds created on the basis of meeting certain performance standards in order to gain pedigree status. Different from purebred breeding, where pedigreeing was based solely on ancestry.

Notes

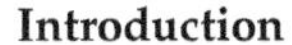

Introduction

1 See John Clay, *My Recollections of Ontario* (Chicago: Private Printing, 1918), 32, 33, 49, 50.
2 L.T.G. Theunissen, *Beauty or Statistics: Practice and Science in Dutch Livestock Breeding 1900–2000* (Toronto: University of Toronto Press, 2020), 48.
3 It has been argued that the entire purebred dog industry was born of commercialism, with dog shows as entertainment. See M. Worboys, J.-M. Strange, and N. Pemberton, *The Invention of the Modern Dog: Breed and Blood in Victorian Britain* (Baltimore: Johns Hopkins University Press, 2018).
4 Sessional Paper 28, Legislature of Ontario (henceforth SP, Ontario), 1898/9, 24–5.
5 M. Denlinger, *The Complete Collie* (Richmond: Denlinger's, 1947, new ed. 1949), 9.
6 The historiography is too vast to list here. A few important examples follow. J. Harwood, *Styles of Scientific Thought: The German Genetics Community, 1900–1933* (Chicago: University of Chicago Press, 1992), and his *Technology's Dilemma: Agricultural Colleges between Science and Practice in Germany 1860–1934* (New York: Peter Lang Publishing Group, 2005); D. Fitzgerald, *Every Farm a Factory* (New Haven: Yale University Press, 2003), and her *The Business of Breeding: Hybrid Corn in Illinois, 1890–1940* (Ithaca: Cornell University Press, 1990); P. Palladino, "Between Craft and Science: Plant Breeding, Mendelian Genetics, and British Universities, 1900–1920," *Technology and Culture* 34 (1993): 300–23; D.B. Paul and B. Kimmelman, "Mendel in America: Theory and Practice, 1900–1919," in *The American Development of Biology*, ed. R. Rainger, K. Benson, and J. Maienschein (Philadelphia: University of Pennsylvania Press, 1988); C. Bonneuil, "Mendelism, Plant Breeding and Experimental Cultures: Agriculture and

the Development of Genetics in France," *Journal of the History of Biology* 39 (2006): 281–308.

7 M.E. Derry, *Art and Science in Breeding: Creating Better Chickens* (Toronto: University of Toronto Press, 2012), and her "Chicken Breeding: The Complex Transition from Traditional to Genetic Methods in the United States," in *Cultivating Knowledge: New Perspectives on the History of Life Sciences and Agriculture*, ed. Sharon Kingsland and Denise Phillips, Archimedes series (New York: Springer, 2015); R. Horowitz, "Making the Chicken of Tomorrow: Reworking Poultry as Commodities and as Creatures, 1945–1990," in *Industrializing Organisms: Introducing Evolutionary History*, ed. S.R. Schrepfer and P. Scranton (London: Routledge, 2004); G.E. Bugos, "Intellectual Property Protection in the American Chicken-Breeding Industry," *Business History Review* 66 (1992): 127–68; G. Sawyer, *The Agribusiness Poultry Industry: A History of Its Development* (New York: Exposition Press, 1971). For Mendelism and the breeding of cattle, see L.T.G. Theunissen, "Breeding without Mendelism: Theory and Practice of Dairy Cattle Breeding in the Netherlands, 1900–1950," *Journal of the History of Biology* 41 (2008): 637–76.

8 See, for example, P. Thurtle, "Harnessing Heredity in Gilded Age America: Middle Class Mores and Industrial Breeding in a Cultural Context," *Journal of the History of Biology* 35 (2002): 33–78, and his *The Emergence of Genetic Rationality: Space, Time, and Transformation in American Biological Science, 1870–1920* (Seattle: University of Washington Press, 2008).

9 A few examples follow. L.T.G. Theunissen, "Breeding for Nobility or Production? Cultures of Dairy Cattle Breeding in the Netherlands, 1945–1995," *Isis* 103 (2012): 278–309, his "The Transformation of the Dutch Farm Horse into a Riding Horse: Livestock Breeding, Science, and Modernization, 1960s–1980s," *Agricultural History* 92 (2018): 24–53, and his *Beauty or Statistics*; M. Derry, *Masterminding Nature: The Breeding of Animals, 1750–2010* (Toronto: University of Toronto Press, 2015); her "Theory and Method: An Analysis of European and American Animal Breeding Practices, 18th to 21st Century," *Agricultural History* 94 (2020): 324–61; her "Genetics, Biotechnology, and Breeding: North American Shorthorn Production in the 21st Century," *Agricultural History* 92 (2018): 54–77; and her "White Collies, Beauty or Genetic Defect: Regulation and Breeding, 1870–2013," *Society and Animals* 28 (2020): 472–88; Jorieke Savelkouls, "A Pure Friesian Is a True Friesian: Innovation and the Persistence of Purity in the Modernization of the Friesian Horse during the Crises of the 1910s and 1960s" and Gianpiero Fumi and Marco Marigliano, "Cattle Breeding in 20th Century Italian Agriculture: From Biometric Selection to Artificial Insemination," both conference papers

given at the European Rural History Conference in Paris, France, 10 September 2019.

10 J. Walton, "The Diffusion of Improved Shorthorn Cattle in Britain during the Eighteenth and Nineteenth Centuries," *Transactions of the Institute of British Geographers* ns 9 (1984): 22–36, and his "Pedigree and the National Cattle Herd circa 1750–1950," *Agricultural History Review* 34 (1986): 149–70; E. Whetham, "The Trade in Pedigree Livestock, 1850–1910," *Agricultural History Review* 27 (1979): 47–50.

11 See, for example, Thurtle, "Harnessing Heredity"; B. Kimmelman, "The American Breeders' Association: Genetics and Eugenics in an Agricultural Context, 1903–1913," *Social Studies of Science* 13 (1983): 163–204. The classics are H. Ritvo, *The Animal Estate* (Cambridge, MA: Harvard University Press, 1987); her *The English and Other Creatures in the Victorian Age* (Cambridge, MA: Harvard University Press, 1987); and her *The Platypus and the Mermaid and Other Figments of the Classifying Imagination* (Cambridge, MA: Harvard University Press, 1997).

1. Animal Breeding Practices and Methods from Roman Times to 1900

1 For a different version of this entire section, see M. Derry, "Theory and Method: An Analysis of European and American Animal Breeding Practices, 18th to 21st Century," *Agricultural History* 94 (2020): 324–61.

2 N. Russell, *Like Engend'ring Like: Heredity and Animal Breeding in Early Modern England* (Cambridge: Cambridge University Press, 1986), 35; J. Lush, *Animal Breeding Plans* (Ames, IA: Collegiate Press, 1937), 146. See also *Marcus Porcius Cato on Agriculture; Marcus Terentius Varro on Agriculture*, rev. H.B. Ash, trans. W.D. Hooper (Cambridge, MA: Harvard University Press, 1934, reprint 1960).

3 N. Russell, *Like Engend'ring Like*, 36.

4 Ibid., 58, 68; V. Orel and R.J. Wood, "Scientific Animal Breeding in Moravia before and after the Discovery of Mendel's Theory," *Quarterly Review of Biology* 75 (2000): 151.

5 N. Russell, *Like Engend'ring Like*, 13. See, as well, S. Müller-Wille and H.J. Rheinberger, *A Cultural History of Heredity* (Chicago: University of Chicago Press, 2012, reprint 2014), for a review of attitudes to heredity up to the end of the eighteenth century.

6 See E. Russell, *Greyhound Nation: A Coevolutionary History of England, 1200–1900* (Cambridge: Cambridge University Press, 2018), 97–101, for a good discussion around environmental breeding.

7 See H.J. Rheinberger and S. Müller-Wille, *The Gene: From Genetics to Postgenomics*, trans. A. Bostanci (Chicago: University of Chicago Press,

2017), chapter 2; Müller-Wille and Rheinberger, *A Cultural History of Heredity*, 28–9, 72–5, 91–2.

8 N. Russell, *Like Engend'ring Like*, 40–1.

9 For more on the subject of environmental impacts on breeding, and especially in relation to colonial importations of animals, see R. Woods, *The Herds Shot around the World: Native Breeds and the British Empire, 1800–1900* (Chapel Hill: University of North Carolina Press, 2017); and S. Swart and G. Bankoff, eds., *Breeds of Empire: The "Invention" of the Horse in Southeast Asia and Southern Africa* (Copenhagen: Nordic Institute of Asian Studies Press, 2007). For attitudes to breeding that existed before the Enlightenment period, see K. Thomas, *Man and the Natural World: Changing Attitudes in England, 1500–1800* (London: Allen Lane, 1983).

10 For Bakewell, see R. Trow-Smith, *A History of British Livestock Husbandry, 1700–1900* (London: Routledge & Kegan Paul, 1959); H.C. Pawson, *Robert Bakewell: Pioneer Livestock Breeder* (London: Crosby Lockwood, 1957) and "Some Agricultural History Salvaged," *Agricultural History Review* 7 (1959): 6–13; R.J. Wood and V. Orel, *Genetic Prehistory in Selective Breeding: A Prelude to Mendel* (Oxford: Oxford University Press, 2001); R.J. Wood, "Robert Bakewell (1725–1795): Pioneer Animal Breeder and His Influence on Charles Darwin," *Folia Mendelianna* 8 (1973): 231–42; D. Wykes, "Robert Bakewell (1725–1795) of Dishley: Farmer and Livestock Improver," *Agricultural History Review* 52 (2004): 38–55.

11 J.V. Beckett, "Note on *Mathew and George Culley: Travel Journals and Letters, 1765–1798*," *English Historical Review* 11 (2003): 803–4; Bakewell to Culley, 8 February 1787, in "The Bakewell Letters," in Pawson, *Robert Bakewell*, 107; G. Mingay, ed. *Arthur Young and His Times* (London: Macmillan Press, 1975), 77–8; S. Sebright, *The Art of Improving Breeds of Domestic Animals* (London: John Harding, 1809).

12 Wood and Orel, *Genetic Prehistory in Selective Breeding*, 89; Sebright, *The Art of Improving Breeds*.

13 Ibid., 10.

14 Wood and Orel, *Genetic Prehistory in Selective Breeding*, 89.

15 I. Glażewska et al., "A New View on Dam Lines in Polish Arabian Horses Based on mtDNA Analysis," *Genetics Selection Evolution* 39 (2007): 609–19; A.T. Bowling et al., "A Pedigree-Based Study of Mitochondrial d-Loop DNA Sequence Variation among Arabian Horses," *Animal Genetics* 31 (2000): 1–7.

16 The literature relating to Thoroughbred horse breeding is extensive. Some valuable sources are the following: R. Cassidy, *Horse People: Thoroughbred Culture in Lexington and Newmarket* (Baltimore: Johns Hopkins University Press, 2007). Ch. 3 (37–53) is the most important. *Tesio: In His Own Words*, trans. M. Burnett (Neenah, WI: Russell Meerdink, 2005). The original

version, F. Tesio's *Puro-Sangue – Animale da Experimento*, was published in 1947 in Milan by Ulrico Hoepli. See also Lady Wentworth, *Thoroughbred Racing Stock* (New York: Charles Scribner's Sons, 1938); F. Mitchell, R. Faversham, and D. Dink, *Racehorse Breeding Theories* (Neenah, WI: Russell Meerdink, 2004); R. Nash, "A Perfect Nicking Pattern," *Humanimalia* 10 (2018): 27–43; M. Derry, *Bred for Perfection: Shorthorn Cattle, Collies, and Arabian Horses since 1800* (Baltimore: Johns Hopkins University Press, 2003), and *Horses in Society: A Story of Breeding and Marketing Culture, 1800–1920* (Toronto: University of Toronto Press, 2006); D. Goodall, *A History of Horse Breeding* (London: Robert Hall, 1977), 33, 145–6, 149; H.H. Barclay, *The Role of the Horse in Human Culture* (London: J.A. Allen, 1980).

17 See P. Kitcher, *In Mendel's Mirror* (Oxford: Oxford University Press, 2003), 63–4.

18 Orel and Wood. "Scientific Animal Breeding in Moravia," 151.

19 Ibid.

20 Ibid.

21 C.J. Bajema, ed., *Artificial Selection and the Development of Evolutionary Theory* (Stroudsburg, PA: Hutchinson Ross Publishing, 1982), 3, 4, 11–12.

22 L.C. Dunn, *A Short History of Genetics: The Development of Some of the Main Lines of Thought, 1864–1939* (New York: McGraw-Hill, 1965), 27–9; Kitcher, *In Mendel's Mirror*, 64. See, as well, Müller-Wille and Rheinberger, *A Cultural History of Heredity*, for more details on early hybridizing and concern with speciation.

23 S. Müller-Wille and V. Orel, "From Linnaean Species to Mendelian Factors: Elements of Hybridism, 1751–1870," *Annals of Science* 64 (2007): 177.

24 Wood and Orel, *Genetic Prehistory in Selective Breeding*.

25 Occasionally breeders utilized the two approaches in attempts to find methods that would deal with both objectives (namely understanding hereditary dynamics and bringing about improvement through homogeneity to certain traits), as was the case with sheep-breeding experiments near Brno, Moravia in the 1830s. See ibid.

26 See A. Sanders, *Short-Horn Cattle: A Series of Historical Sketches, Memoirs and Records of the Breed and Its Development in the United States and Canada* (Chicago: Sanders, 1900), 14, 31, 34–5, 37–9, 44, 75, 81–5; S. Wright, "Mendelian Analysis of the Pure Bred Breeds of Livestock, Part 2, The Duchess Family of Shorthorns As Bred by Thomas Bates," *Journal of Heredity* 14 (1923): 339–48; C.J. Bates, *Thomas Bates and the Kirklevington Shorthorns: A Contribution to the History of Pure Durham Cattle* (Newcastle upon Tyne: Robert Redpath, 1897).

27 After a dinner party in 1820, Lord Althorp, who greatly admired Bates's cattle, turned to a friend and said: "A wonderful, wonderful man! He

might become anything – Prime Minister – if he would not talk so much." Quoted in Sanders, *Short-Horn Cattle*, 69, 80.

28 See, for example, *Farmer's Advocate*, January 1876, 13; February 1876, 27; March 1876, 46; 8 December 1910, 1927–8; *Farming World and Canadian Farm and Home*, 1 January 1906, 161. See Sessional Paper 13, Legislature of Ontario (henceforth SP, Ontario), 1875–6, 31–2; SP 12, Ontario, 1877, 48.

29 See, for example, B. Kimmelman, "The American Breeders' Association: Genetics and Eugenics in an Agricultural Context, 1903–1913," *Social Studies of Science* 13 (1983): 163–204.

30 Müller-Wille and Rheinberger, *A Cultural History of Heredity*, 80.

31 Ibid., 134.

32 C. Darwin, *On the Origin of Species* (London: John Murray, 1859), 13. The literature on Darwin and his knowledge of how heredity worked is extensive. See, for example, S.E. Kingsland, "The Battling Botanist: Daniel Trembly MacDougal, Mutation Theory, and the Rise of Experimental Evolutionary Biology in America, 1900–1912," *Isis* 82 (1991): 484–5; and R. Olby, *Origins of Mendelism*, 2nd ed. (Chicago: University of Chicago Press, 1985), 40–7.

33 D.B. Paul and B.A. Kimmelman, "Mendel in America: Theory and Practice, 1900–1919," in R. Rainger et al., eds., *The American Development of Biology* (Philadelphia: University of Pennsylvania Press, 1988), 289; B.A. Matz, "Crafting Heredity: The Art and Science of Livestock Breeding in the United States and Germany, 1860–1914," PhD thesis, Yale University, December 2011, 169–75, 207.

34 L.T.G. Theunissen, "Knowledge Is Power: Hugo de Vries on Science, Heredity and Social Progress," *British Journal for the History of Science* 27 (1994): 293, 301, 304.

35 Kingsland, "The Battling Botanist," 489–93.

36 Paul and Kimmelman, "Mendel in America," 289, 293; USDA, Yearbook of Agriculture, "Better Plants and Animals," Part 1 (1936), 469; L. Carlson, "Forging His Own Path: William Jasper Spillman and Progressive Era Breeding and Genetics," *Agricultural History* 79 (2005): 50, 52, 53, 58.

37 Matz, "Crafting Heredity," 212–16.

38 J.A. Secord, "Nature's Fancy: Charles Darwin and the Breeding of Pigeons," *Isis* 72 (1981): 166–71, 174, 177. For more on Darwin's interest in artificial selection, see S.G. Alter, "The Advantages of Obscurity: Charles Darwin's Negative Inference from the Histories of Domestic Breeds," *Annals of Science* 64 (2007): 235–50; R.A. Richards, "Darwin and the Inefficacy of Artificial Selection," *Studies in History and Philosophy of Science* 28 (1997): 75–97; S.G. Sterrett, "Darwin's Analogy between Artificial and Natural Selection: How Does It Go?" *Studies in History and Philosophy of Biological and Biomedical Sciences* 33 (2002): 151–68; L.T. Evans,

"Darwin's Use of the Analogy between Artificial and Natural Selection," *Journal of the History of Biology* 17 (1984): 113–40; J.F. Cornell, "Analogy and Technology in Darwin's Vision of Nature," *Journal of the History of Biology* 17 (1984): 303–44; H.J. Rheinberger and P. McLaughlin, "Darwin's Experimental Natural History," *Journal of the History of Biology* 17 (1984): 345–68; and L.T.G. Theunissen, "Darwin and His Pigeons: The Analogy between Artificial and Natural Selection Revisited," *Journal of the History of Biology* 45 (2012): 179–212.

39 Theunissen, "Darwin and His Pigeons."

40 For more on Galton's law, see P. Froggatt and N.C. Nevin, "Galton's 'Law of Ancestral Heredity': Its Influence on the Early Development of Human Genetics," *History of Science* 10 (1971): 1–27; M. Bulmer, "Galton's Law of Ancestral Heredity," *Heredity* 81 (1998): 579–85; N.W. Gillham, "Evolution by Jumps: Francis Galton and William Bateson and the Mechanism of Evolutionary Change," *Genetics* 159 (2001): 1383–92; P. Froggatt and N.C. Nevin, "The 'Law of Ancestral Heredity' and the Mendelian-Ancestrian Controversy in England, 1889–1906," *Journal of Medical Genetics* 8 (1971): 1–36.

41 In its first issue, Galton stated: "The primary object of Biometry is to afford material that shall be exact enough for the discovery of incipient changes in evolution which are too small to be otherwise apparent." M. Bulmer, *Francis Galton: Pioneer of Heredity and Biometry* (Baltimore: Johns Hopkins University Press, 2003), 299.

42 J.L. Lush, "Genetics and Animal Breeding," in Dunn, ed., *Genetics in the 20th Century*, 494.

43 N.R. Gillham, *A Life of Sir Francis Galton: From African Exploration to the Birth of Eugenics* (Oxford: Oxford University Press, 2001), 9.

44 Ibid.; W.G. Hill, ed., *Quantitative Genetics: Part I, Explanation and Analysis of Continuous Variation* (New York: Van Nostrand Reinhold, 1984), 9, 10. For examples of Pearson's work on the subject, see his "On the Systematic Fitting of Curves to Measurements and Observations: Part I," *Biometrika* 1 (1902): 265–303, "On the Systematic Fitting of Curves to Measurements and Observations: Part II," *Biometrika* 2 (1902): 1–23, and "On the Systematic Fitting of Curves to Measurements and Observations: Part I," *Biometrika* 1 (1902): 266.

45 M. Worboys, J.-M. Strange, and N. Pemberton, *The Invention of the Modern Dog: Breed and Blood in Victorian Britain* (Baltimore: Johns Hopkins University Press, 2018), 169.

46 Francis Galton, "The Average Contribution of Each Several Ancestor to the Total Heritage of the Offspring," *Proceedings of the Royal Society* 61 (1897): 402, 403.

47 Ibid., 408.

48 See, for example, *Breeder's Gazette*, 27 June 1888, 642; 15 August 1888, 154; 2 March 1892, 173.
49 *American Poultry Journal*, August 1910, 976–7. See, as well, I.K. Felch, *Poultry Culture: How to Raise, Mate and Judge Thoroughbred Fowl* (Chicago: Donohue, Henneberry, 1902).
50 W.D. Termohlen, "Past History and Future Developments," *Poultry Science* 47 (1968): 12; *American Poultry Journal*, August 1911, 1268. A particularly clear description of Felch's inbreeding strategies and his chart appeared in an agricultural circular published in 1911 in Alberta: "Practical Poultry Keeping," Poultry Bulletin 2, Alberta Department of Agriculture, 1911, 73.
51 *American Poultry Journal*, August 1911, 1268.
52 I.K. Felch, *The Breeding and Management of Poultry* (Hyde Park, NY: Norfolk County Press, 1877), 47.
53 An example might be seen in *American Poultry Journal*, November 1908, 736.
54 *American Poultry Journal*, December 1922, 1112–13. See ibid., November 1906, 910, as well.
55 Felch, *The Breeding and Management of Poultry*, 47.
56 Worboys, Strange, and Pemberton, *The Invention of the Modern Dog*, 169.

2. Mendelism, Quantitative Genetics, and Animal Breeding, 1900–2000

1 See H.J. Rheinberger and S. Müller-Wille, *The Gene: From Genetics to Postgenomics*, trans. Adam Bostanci (Chicago: University of Chicago Press, 2017), ch. 2.
2 D.C. Warren, "A Half Century of Advances in the Genetics and Breeding Improvement of Poultry," *Poultry Science* 37 (1958): 3–5.
3 Geneticist Wilhelm Johanssen recognized the value of pure breeding lines – commonly followed by the practical breeders – for scientific experiments, but he still emphasized the hybridizing method. In the decade after the rediscovery of Mendel's laws, he believed Mendelist experiments followed one of two procedures: working with pure lines only or hybridizing by using those pure lines. S. Müller-Wille and H.J. Rheinberger, *A Cultural History of Heredity* (Chicago: University of Chicago Press, 2012, reprint 2014), 128. See also W. Johanssen, "The Genotype Conception of Heredity," *American Naturalist* 45 (1911): 129–59.
4 *Collie Folio*, January 1908, 21–2.
5 Ibid., September 1911, 308.
6 Ibid., June 1912, 207.
7 Ibid., 208.

8 See *American Poultry Journal*, May 1913, 847 for Pearl's comments in the Maine Experiment Station Bulletin 305, 1913, 388. See, as well, K. Cooke, "From Science to Practice, or Practice to Science? Chickens and Eggs in Raymond Pearl's Agricultural Breeding Research, 1907–1916," *Isis* 88 (1997): 62–86; M.E. Derry, *Art and Science in Breeding: Creating Better Chickens* (Toronto: University of Toronto Press, 2012), 99–105.

9 *American Poultry Journal*, April 1913, 672.

10 Ibid., May 1913, 847.

11 *American Breeders' Magazine* 3 (1912): 271. See also W.E. Castle, *Heredity in Relation to Evolution and Animal Breeding* (New York: D. Appleton and Company, 1911); W.E. Castle, "Pure Lines and Selection," *Journal of Heredity* 5 (1914): 93–7.

12 D.F. Jones, "Dominance of Linked Factors as a Means of Accounting for Heterosis," *Genetics* 2 (1917): 471.

13 D. Fitzgerald, *The Business of Breeding: Hybrid Corn in Illinois, 1890–1940* (Ithaca: Cornell University Press, 1990), 55; and J.R. Kloppenburg, *First the Seed: The Political Economy of Plant Biotechnology, 1492–2000* (Cambridge: Cambridge University Press, 1988), 99.

14 Fitzgerald, *The Business of Breeding*.

15 G. Sawyer, *The Agribusiness Poultry Industry: A History of Its Development* (New York: Exposition Press, 1971), 112; E.L. Schapsmeier and F.H. Schapsmeier, *Henry A. Wallace of Iowa: The Agrarian Years, 1910–1940* (Ames: Iowa State University Press, 1968), 21, 27, 28.

16 A great deal has been written about chicken breeding. For example, see the following: I.K. Felch, *The Breeding and Management of Poultry* (Hyde Park, NY: Norfolk County Press, 1877), 47. See as well I.K. Felch, *Poultry Culture: How to Raise, Mate and Judge Thoroughbred Fowl* (Chicago: Donohue, Henneberry, 1902); Sawyer, *The Agribusiness Poultry Industry*; O.A. Hanke, ed., *American Poultry History, 1823–1973* (Madison, WI: American Poultry History Society, 1974); F.A. Hayes and G.T. Klein, *Poultry Breeding Applied* (Mount Morris, IL: Watt Publishing Company, 1952), 192–5; D.C. Warren, "Techniques of Hybridization of Poultry," *Poultry Science* 29 (1950); A.L. Hagedoorn and G. Sykes, *Poultry Breeding: Theory and Practice* (London: Crosby Lockwood & Son, 1953); Derry, *Art and Science in Breeding*; Warren, "A Half Century of Advances in the Genetics and Breeding Improvement of Poultry"; R. Horowitz, "Making the Chicken of Tomorrow: Reworking Poultry as Commodities and as Creatures, 1945–1990," in *Industrializing Organisms: Introducing Evolutionary History*, ed. S.R. Schaefer and P. Scranton (London: Routledge, 2004); G.E. Bugos, "Intellectual Property Protection in the American Chicken-Breeding Industry," *Business History Review* 66 (1992): 127–68.

17 The chicken meat, or broiler, industry is a separate story involving not just hybridizing for biological locks but also a structural change, which brought about vertical integration of the industry from breeder to producer to the end marketers of meat. Integration would play a role in the egg industry as well. See, in particular, Horowitz, "Making the Chicken of Tomorrow"; Sawyer, *The Agribusiness Poultry Industry*; Derry, *Art and Science in Breeding*.

18 By the 1970s, inbreeding/hybridizing began to affect the pig industry – especially in Britain and continental Europe – via companies who used the method to produce boars. While the situation did not match the chicken industry's experience, the companies – who sold breeding rights on hybrid boars – relied on the same biological lock to protect their interests. See P. Brassley, "Cutting across Nature? The History of Artificial Insemination in Pigs in the United Kingdom," *Studies in History and Philosophy of Biological and Biomedical Sciences* 38 (2007): 444–5, 452, 458–9. For more on pig breeding, see J. Webb's "Animal Breeding Practice" in W.G. Hill and T.F.C. Mackay, eds, *Evolution and Animal Breeding: Reviews on Molecular and Quantitative Approaches in Honour of Alan Robertson* (Wallingford, UK: C.A.B. International, 1989), 195–7.

19 See R.W. Touchberry, "Crossbreeding Effects in Dairy Cattle: The Illinois Experiment, 1949–1969," *Journal of Dairy Science* 75 (1992): 640–67; J.L. Lush, "Dairy Cattle Genetics," ibid. 39 (1956): 693–4; J.M. White et al., "Dairy Cattle Improvement and Genetics," ibid. 64 (1981): 1310, 1311; R.C. Laben et al., "Some Effects of Inbreeding and Evidence of Heterosis through Outcrossing in a Holstein-Friesian Herd," ibid. 38 (1955): 525–35; F.R. Allaire et al., "Specific Combing Abilities among Dairy Sires," ibid. 48 (1965): 1096, 1099; R.C. Beckett et al., "Specific and General Combining Abilities for Production and Reproduction among Lines of Holstein Cattle," ibid. 62 (1979): 613, 619.

20 White et al., "Dairy Cattle Improvement and Genetics," 1310.

21 Series 1, box 11, file 4, Shaver Collection, Archival and Special Collections, University of Guelph. Also Derry, *Art and Science in Breeding*, 196–7.

22 P. Henlein, "Cattle Driving from the Ohio Valley, 1800–1850," *Agricultural History* 28 (1954): 94; "Shifting Range-Feeding Patterns in the Ohio Valley before 1860," ibid. 31 (1957): 1–11; "Cattle Kingdom in the Ohio Valley: The Beef Cattle Industry in the Ohio Valley, 1783–1860" (PhD diss; University of Wisconsin, 1957); E.M. Ensminger, *Beef Cattle Science* (Danville: Interstate Printers and Publishers, 1987); M.E. Derry, *Ontario's Cattle Kingdom: Purebred Breeders and Their World, 1870–1920* (Toronto: University of Toronto Press, 2001); T. Jordan, *North American Cattle Ranching Frontiers: Origins, Diffusion, and Differentiation*, Histories of the American Frontier (Albuquerque: University of New Mexico Press,

1993); J. Whitacker, *Feedlot Empire: Beef Cattle Feeding in Illinois and Iowa, 1840–1900* (Ames: Iowa State University Press, 1975), 55, 64, 82; J.H. Von Thünen, *Der Isolieerte Staatt*, trans. C. Wartenburg (Oxford: Pergamon Press, 1966).

23 See E. Mayr and W.B. Provine, *The Evolutionary Synthesis: Perspectives on the Unification of Biology* (Cambridge, MA: Harvard University Press, 1980).

24 W.G. Hill, "Applications of Population Genetics to Animal Breeding, from Wright and Lush to Genomic Prediction," *Genetics* 196 (2014): 1.

25 J. Lush, "Genetics and Animal Breeding," in *Genetics in the 20th Century*, ed. L.C. Dunn (New York: Macmillan Company, 1951), 494–5; Lush, *Animal Breeding Plans* (Ames, IA: Collegiate Press, 1937), 145.

26 Ibid., 181.

27 W.G. Hill, "Applications of Population Genetics to Animal Breeding," 2; Lush, *Animal Breeding Plans*; A.B. Chapman, "Jay Lawrence Lush 1896–1982: A Brief Biography," *Journal of American Science* 69 (1991): 2674; A. Freeman, "Genetic Statistics in Animal Breeding," in *Proceedings* of the Animal Breeding and Genetic Symposium in Honor of Dr. Jay L. Lush (American Society of Animal Science and American Dairy Science Association, 1972), 6; L. Ollivier, "Jay Lush: Reflections on the Past," *Lohmann Information* 43 (2008): 3–12; G.E. Dickerson, "Inbreeding and Heterosis in Animals," in *Proceedings*, 54.

28 W.G. Hill, "Applications of Population Genetics to Animal Breeding", 2; W.G. Hill, ed., *Quantitative Genetics: Part I, Explanation and Analysis of Continuous Variation* (New York: Van Nostrand Reinhold Company, 1984), 16; W.G. Hill, ed., *Quantitative Genetics: Part II, Selection* (New York: Van Nostrand Reinhold Company, 1984), 1, 2, 10, 11, 12; M. Lynch and B. Walsh, *Genetics and Analysis of Quantitative Traits* (Sunderland, MA: Sinauer Associates, 1998); E.P. Cunningham, *Quantitative Genetic Theory and Livestock Improvement* (Armidale, NSW: University of New England, 1979).

29 W. Provine, *Sewall Wright and Evolutionary Biology* (Chicago: University of Chicago Press, 1986), 138–9, 140, 141, and *The Origins of Theoretical Population Genetics* (Chicago: University of Chicago Press, 1971), 160–1; J.F. Crow, "Sewall Wright's Place in Twentieth-Century Biology," *Journal of the History of Biology* 23 (1990): 63; S. Wright, "The Effects of Inbreeding and Crossbreeding on Guinea Pigs," Bulletin 1090, United States Department of Agriculture, 1922; and *Systems of Mating and Other Papers* (Ames: Iowa State College Press, 1958), which contains reprints of his "Systems of Mating," *Genetics* 6 (1921): 111–78, "Evolution in Mendelian Populations," ibid. 16 (1931): 97–159, "Correlation and Causation," *Journal of Agricultural Research* 20 (1921): 557–85, and "The Method of Path Coefficients," *Annals of Mathematical Statistics* 5 (1934): 161–215.

30 R.A. Fisher, "The Correlation between Relatives on the Supposition of Mendelian Inheritance," *Transactions of the Royal Society of Edinburgh* 52 (1918): 399–433. See, as well, J.E. Box, *R.A. Fisher: The Life of a Scientist* (New York: Wiley, 1978).

31 W.G. Hill, "Applications of Population Genetics to Animal Breeding," 1–16. Many considered Lush's paper "Family Merit and Individual Merit as Bases for Selection," *American Naturalist* 81 (1947): 241–61, to be his best.

32 Animal genetics would in turn serve studies of evolution. See W.G. Hill and M. Kirkpatrick, "What Animal Breeding Has Taught Us about Evolution," *Annual Review of Ecology, Evolution, and Systematics* 41 (2010): 1–19.

33 Lush, "Genetics and Animal Breeding," 506–7.

34 Snedecor's most significant work was *Statistical Methods Applied to Experiments in Agriculture and Biology*, published in 1937. See D. Gianola et al., eds., *Advances in Statistical Methods for Genetic Improvement of Livestock* (Berlin: Springer-Verlag, 1990), 4.

35 L.N. Hazel, "The Genetic Basis for Constructing Selection Indexes," *Genetics* 28 (1943): 476–90; Hazel et al., "The Selection Index – Then, Now, and for the Future," *Journal of Dairy Science* 77 (1994): 3236–51; C.R. Henderson, *Applications of Linear Models in Animal Breeding* (Guelph, ON: University of Guelph, 1984) (online: cgil.uoguelph.ca/pub/Henderson.html); "Young Sire Selection for Commercial Artificial Insemination," *Journal of Dairy Science* 47 (1964): 439–46; "General Flexibility of Linear Model Techniques for Sire Evaluation," ibid. 57 (1974): 963–72; and "Historical Overview," in Gianola et al., eds., *Advances in Statistical Methods*.

36 D. Falconer, "Quantitative Genetics in Edinburgh, 1947–1980," *Genetics* 133 (1993); A. Robertson, "Crossbreeding Experiments with Dairy Cattle (A Review)," *Animal Breeding Abstracts* 17 (1949): 201, and his "Inbreeding in Artificial Selection Programmes," *Genetic Research* 2 (1961): 189–94, and with J.M. Rendel, "The Use of Progeny Testing with Artificial Insemination in Dairy Cattle," *Journal of Genetics* 50 (1950): 21–31.

37 R. Vishwanath, "Artificial Insemination: The State of the Art," *Theriogenology* 59 (2003); H.A. Herman, *Improving Cattle by the Millions: NAAB and the Development and Worldwide Application of Artificial Insemination* (Columbia: University of Missouri Press, 1981); S. Wilmot, "From 'Public Service' to Artificial Insemination: Animal Breeding Science and Reproductive Research in Early 20th Century Britain," *Studies in History and Philosophy of Biological and Biomedical Sciences* 38 (2007); R.H. Foote, "The Artificial Insemination Industry," in B.J. Brackett et al., eds., *New Technologies in Animal Breeding* (New York: Academic

Press, 1981), 14; and his "The History of Artificial Insemination: Selected Notes and Notables," *Journal of Animal Science* 80 (2002); D.A. Funk, "Major Advances in Globalization and Consolidation of the Artificial Insemination Industry," *Journal of Dairy Science* 89 (2006).

38 X. David et al., "International Genomic Cooperation: EuroGenomics Significantly Improves Reliability of Genomic Evaluations," *Interbull Bulletin* 41, 77–8, Interbull Workshop, Paris 2010. See, as well, R. Dassonneville et al., "Effect of Imputing Markers from a Low-Density Chip on the Reliability of Genomic Breeding Values in Holstein Populations," *Journal of Dairy Science* 94 (2011): 3679–86; A. Loberg et al., "Interbull Survey on the Use of Genomic Evaluations," *Proceedings of the Interbull International Workshop*, Bulletin 38 (2009): 3, 4, 5, 6, 9.

39 F.J. Arnold, "Fifty Years of DHIA Work," *Journal of Dairy Science* 39 (1956): 793; D.E. Voelker, "Dairy Herd Improvement Associations," ibid. 64 (1981); L.W. Morley, "Dairy Cattle Breed Associations," ibid., 39 (1956).

40 For more on the dairy industry, see S. McMurry, *Transforming Rural America: Dairying Families and Agricultural Change, 1820–1885* (Baltimore: Johns Hopkins University Press, 1995); E.E. Lampard, *The Rise of the Dairy Industry in Wisconsin: A Study of Agricultural Change, 1820–1920* (Madison: State Historical Society of Wisconsin, 1963); Morley, "Dairy Cattle Breed Associations"; B. Orland, "Turbo-Cows: Producing a Competitive Animal in the Nineteenth and Early Twentieth Centuries," in *Industrializing Organisms: Introducing Evolutionary History*, ed. S.R. Schrepfer and P. Scranton (London: Routledge, 2004); Arnold, "Fifty Years of DHIA Work," 792; Voelker, "Dairy Herd Improvement Associations"; G.M. Trout, "Fifty Years of the American Dairy Science Association," *Journal of Dairy Science* 39 (1956).

41 Vishwanath, "Artificial Insemination," 571, 572.

42 I.M. Lerner and H. Donald, *Modern Developments in Animal Breeding* (London and New York: Academic Press, 1966), 170, 171, 178–9, 185.

43 For more on the beef industry, see B.L. Golden et al., "Milestones in Beef Cattle Genetic Evaluations," *Journal of Animal Science* 87 (2009): E3–10; A.L. Eller, "A Look Back at BIF History," *Proceedings* of Annual Beef Improvement Federation Symposium (2007): 10–14; R.M. Bourdon, "Shortcomings of Current Genetic Evaluation Systems," *Journal of Animal Science* 76 (1998): 2308–23. Particularly important are the Proceedings of the Beef Improvement Federation Conferences. These articles are available on the website: www.beefimprovement.org/proceedings.html. (If a 404 error appears, ignore this. Go to "Convention" on the menu and press "Proceedings." All articles by year will be there.)

44 M. Derry, "Genetics, Biotechnology, and Breeding: North American Shorthorn Production in the 21st Century," *Agricultural History* 92 (Winter

2018). CHAROLAIS CATTLE (IMPORT), House of Commons Debates, 10 April 1963, vol. 675, cc 1437–48, http://hansard.millbanksystems.com/commons/1963/apr/10/charolais-cattle-import; and http://simmental-sbl.blogspot.ca/2011/12/about-this-blog.html; http://simmental-sbl.blogspot.ca/, accessed 30 October 2015; Don Vaniman, executive secretary of the American Simmental Association, *Simmental Shield,* August 1974, 119–22.

45 G. MacEwan, *Highlights of Shorthorn History* (Winnipeg: Hignell Printing, 1982), 197–8.

46 Ibid., 198–9.

47 F. Mitchell, R. Faversham, and D. Dink, *Racehorse Breeding Theories* (Neenah, WI: Russell Meerdink, 2004), 273–306, 191–236; Tesio, *Tesio: In His Own Words*, trans. M. Burnett (Neenah, WI: Russell Meerdink Company, 2005); R. Cassidy, *Horse People: Thoroughbred Culture in Lexington and Newmarket* (Baltimore: Johns Hopkins University Press, 2007), 37–53.

48 W.G. Hill, "Applications of Population Genetics to Animal Breeding," 12.

49 O. Kempthorne, "An Overview of the Field of Quantitative Genetics," in E. Pollak et al., eds., *Proceedings of the International Conference on Quantitative Genetics* (Ames: Iowa State University Press, 1977), 48

50 See Ann Millán Gasca, "The Biology of Numbers: The Correspondence of Vito Volterra on Mathematical Biology," in *The Biology of Numbers: The Correspondence of Vito Volterra on Mathematical Biology*, ed. G. Israel and Ann Millán Gasca, Science Networks. Historical Studies 26 (Berlin: Birkauser Verlag, 2002), 1–54; and S.E. Kingsland, "Mathematical Figments, Biological Facts: Population Ecology in the Thirties," *Journal of the History of Biology* 19 (1986): 235–56.

3. Animal Breeding in the Age of Molecular Genetics, Genomics, and Epigenetics, 1990–2020

1 Recombinant DNA technology opened up the possibility of assessing genes at the DNA level, and laid the basis for genomics.

2 O. Kempthorne, "Introduction," in E. Pollak et al., eds., *Proceedings of the International Conference on Quantitative Genetics* (Ames: Iowa State University Press, 1977), 5–9, 10. See as well E.P. Cunningham, *Quantitative Genetic Theory and Livestock Improvement* (Armidale, NSW: University of New England, 1979), 9; M. Lynch and B. Walsh, *Genetics and Analysis of Quantitative Traits* (Sunderland, MA: Sinauer Associates, 1998), 390.

3 O. Kempthorne, "Introduction," *Proceedings*, 10–11.

4 R.E. Comstock, "Quantitative Genetics and the Design of Breeding Programs," *Proceedings*, 705–18.

5 D.L. Harris, "Past, Present and Potential Contributions of Quantitative Genetics to Applied Animal Breeding," *Proceedings*, 588.
6 See Bruno Latour, *Science in Action* (Cambridge, MA: Harvard University Press, 1987) for the classic discussion concerning black box thinking and black box theory in various disciplines.
7 R. Lewontin, "The Relevance of Molecular Biology to Plant and Animal Breeding," *Proceedings*, 56.
8 Ibid.
9 Ibid.
10 Book review of *Proceedings* by P.E. Smouse, in *American Journal of Human Genetics*, 31 (1979): 754.
11 See A. Robertson, "Molecular Biology and Animal Breeding," *Annales de Génétique et de Sélection animale* 2 (1970): 393–402.
12 QTL (quantitiative trait loci) are the loci of genetic material proven to relate to productive traits in livestock. The loci can be genes, or simply stretches of DNA that do not code for protein (meaning they do not specify how the protein used to build cells in the body will develop and function) if these stretches are known to be close to the genes that regulate traits sought after. B.J. Hayes, "QTL Mapping, MAS, and Genomic Selection," Short Course, *Animal Breeding and Genetics* (Department of Animal Science, Iowa State University, 2007), 55, https://www.ans.iastate.edu/research/animal-breeding-and-genetics/short-course/past-short-courses/summer-2007, accessed June 2021. For plants and QTL, see K.R. Lambey and M. Lee, "Quantitative Genetics, Molecular Markers, and Plant Improvement," *Focused Plant Improvement: Towards Responsible and Sustainable Agriculture. Proceedings of the 10th Australian Plant Breeding Conference*, 1993.
13 See C.W. Beattie, "Development of Detailed Microsatellite Linkage Maps in Livestock," in *Biotechnology's Role in the Genetic Improvement of Farm Animals*, ed. R.H. Miller et al. (Beltsville Symposia in Agricultural Research, American Society of Animal Science, 1996), 52, 57; J.I. Weller, "Introduction to QTL Detection and Marker-Assisted Selection," in ibid., 259, 261, 261.
14 See W. Barendse, "Development and Commercialization of a Genetic Marker for Marbling of Beef in Cattle: A Case Study," in M. Rothschild and S. Newman, eds., *Intellectual Property Rights in Animal Breeding and Genetics* (New York: CABI Publishing, 2002), 197–212.
15 Eenennaam et al., "Validation of Commercial DNA Tests for Quantitative Beef Quality Traits," *Journal of Animal Science* 85 (2007): 899.
16 J.M. Lapointe, S. Lachance, and D.J. Steffen, "Tibial Hemimelia, Meningocele, and Abdominal Hernia in Shorthorn Cattle," *Veterinary Pathology* 37, no. 5 (2000): 508–11. The TH situation in Shorthorns soon

proved to be more complicated. Descendants of TKA Outcast, a bull born in 2001, could inherit a form of deletion much larger than the one in the line from the Improver bull. The Outcast one overlapped the Improver deletion in gene *ALX4* and involved three other genes. Calves are affected when they inherit both the Improver and the Outcast deletion. Known as "compound heterozygotes," these calves are defective in the same way as calves homozygous for the Improver deletion. The Outcast mutation is, however, rare. See B.K. Whitlock, L. Kaiser, and H.S. Maxwell, "Heritable Bovine Fetal Abnormalities," *Top Stock Magazine*, March 2016, 546.

17 *High Plains Journal*, 8 December 2008, http://www.hpj.com/archives/shorthorn-mutation-was-beginning-of-current-genetic-research/article_217fb2f4-6646-5bc8-a972–7e4a80d58f56.html, accessed 26 October 2017.

18 Star Search IV catalogue, 2006, printed in *Shorthorn Country*, August 2006; Star Search V, 2007, printed in ibid., August 2007; Star Search VI, 2008, printed in ibid., August 2008.

19 Ibid.

20 For example, see RC Show Cattle catalogue for the 22nd Early Bird Auction, 2014.

21 http://www.steerplanet.com/bb/the-big-show/potential-genetic-defect-in-shorthorn-cattle/540/, accessed 20 September 2014; http://www.steerplanet.com/bb/the-big-show/problem-with-club-calf-industry-thoughts-please/50/?wap2, accessed 10 November 2014.

22 Whitlock, Kaiser, and Maxwell, "Heritable Bovine Fetal Abnormalities," 546.

23 http://www.steerplanet.com/bb/the-big-show/pha-and-th-bulls/5/?wap2, accessed 10 September 2015; http://www.steerplanet.com/bb/the-big-show/flushing-thc-to-a-thc/, accessed 23 January 2015.

24 http://www.steerplanet.com/bb/the-big-show/potential-genetic-defect-in-shorthorn-cattle/585/, accessed 4 November 2014.

25 Beef Shorthorn Society TH Policy, http://www.beefshorthorn.org/index.php/the-breed/beef-shorthorn/policy-regarding-th, accessed 3 October 2015.

26 A.J. Clarke, ed., *Animal Breeding: Technology for the 21st Century* (Amsterdam: Harwood, 1998), 7.

27 G.E. Pollott, "Bioinformatical Genetics – Opening the Black Box of Quantitative Genetics," *Proceedings of the World Congress on Genetics Applied to Livestock Production* (2006): 23.21; D. Habier, R. Fernando, and D. Garrick, "Genomic BLUP Decoded: A Look into the Black Box of Genomic Prediction," *Genetics* 194 (2013): 597–607; W.G. Hill, "Applications of Population Genetics to Animal Breeding, from Wright and Lush to Genomic Prediction," ibid. 196 (2014): 9.

28 B. Walsh, "Quantitative Genetics, Version 3.0: Where Have We Gone since 1987 and Where Are We Headed?" *Genetica* 136 (2009): 215.
29 The DNA molecule forms a double helix, in which two long chains of nucleotide subunits twist around each other, forming a right-handed helix. There are four bases in the chains – A (adenine), T (thymine), G (guanine), or C (cytosine). Where one strand has an A, the other has a T, and where one has a G, the other has a C. Species differ only by the sequence of the A, G, T, and C nucleotides.
30 *Hoard's Dairyman*, July 2008, 472.
31 The seminal paper behind genomic breeding is T.H.E. Meuwissen et al. in "Prediction of Total Genetic Value Using Genome-Wide Marker Maps," *Genetics* 157 (2001): 1819–29; W.G. Hill, "Applications of Population Genetics to Animal Breeding."
32 J. van der Werf, "Animal Breeding and the Black Box of Biology," *Journal of Animal Breeding and Genetics* 124 (2007): 101.
33 J.W. Keele et al., "Databases and Information Systems Needed for Maps and Marker-Assisted Selection," in *Biotechnology's Role in the Genetic Improvement of Farm Animals*, ed. R.H. Miller et al. (Beltsville Symposia in Agricultural Research, American Society of Animal Science, 1996), 300.
34 S.S. Moore, "The Bovine Genome Sequence – Will It Live Up to the Promise?" *Journal of Animal Science and Genetics* 126 (2009): 257; G.R. Wiggans, "Selection of Single-Nucleotide Polymorphisms and Quality of Genotypes Used in Genomic Evaluation of Dairy Cattle in the United States and Canada," *Journal of Dairy Science* 92 (2009): 3431.
35 See W.G. Hill, "Applications of Population Genetics to Animal Breeding," 1–16; M. Derry, *Masterminding Nature: The Breeding of Animals, 1750–2010* (Toronto: University of Toronto Press, 2015).
36 *Nature* 496 (2013): 420.
37 See the last chapter of H.J. Rheinberger and S. Müller-Wille, *The Gene: From Genetics to Postgenomics*, trans. Adam Bostanci (Chicago: University of Chicago Press, 2017), for an assessment of epigenetics.
38 For example, ibid.; Clemens Driessen, "Deliberating with Crispr Creatures – When Bioethics Becomes a Matter of More-Than-Human/Cultural Geography," unpublished paper, Uppsala University, Sweden, May 2018. See S. Richardson and H. Stevens, eds., *Postgenomics* (Durham, NC: Duke University Press, 2015). For CRISPR Cas 9, see A.C. Komor et al., "CRISPR-Based Technologies for the Manipulation of Eukaryotic Genomes," *Cell* 168 (2017); Yue Mei, "Recent Progress in CRISPR/Cas9 Technology," *Journal of Genetics and Genomics* 43 (2016): 63–75; "Gene Editing Research Review," https://www.illumina.com/content/dam/illumina-marketing/documents/products/research_reviews/publication-review-gene-editing-research.pdf, accessed 14 June 2018).

4. Specialization for Purpose and Animal Breeding

1 M. Worboys, J.-M. Strange, and N. Pemberton, *The Invention of the Modern Dog: Breed and Blood in Victorian Britain* (Baltimore: Johns Hopkins University Press, 2018), 37–9.
2 E. Russell, in his *Greyhound Nation: A Coevolutionary History of England, 1200–1900* (Cambridge: Cambridge University Press, 2018), provides a detailed description of environmental breeding in chapter 2. Most other sources only offer generalities.
3 J. Walsh (Stonehenge), *The Greyhound in 1864: Breeding, Rearing, and Training of Greyhounds* (London: Longman, Green, Longman, Roberts & Green, 1864), 207–9.
4 *Kennel Gazette* (British), November 1883, 489.
5 See the section "Three Niches, Three Populations" in E. Russell's *Greyhound Nation*. This book gives a wonderfully detailed description of Greyhound breeding, the developments that related to the sport of racing and showing the dogs under the Kennel Club system, and ways people used and worked with the dogs over centuries.
6 Worboys, Strange, and Pemberton, *The Invention of the Modern Dog*, 78.
7 For more detail on the beauty/utility issue, see M. Derry, "Chicken Breeding: The Complex Transition from Traditional to Genetic Methods in the United States," in *Cultivating Knowledge: New Perspectives on the History of Life Sciences and Agriculture*, ed. Sharon Kingsland and Denise Phillips, Archimedes Series (New York: Springer, 2015), and her *Art and Science in Breeding: Creating Better Chickens* (Toronto: University of Toronto Press, 2012).
8 *Farmer's Advocate*, September 1876, 177.
9 *American Poultry Journal*, February 1925, 341.
10 E. Brown, *Races of Domestic Poultry* (London: Edward Arnold, 1906), 203, 204.
11 *American Poultry Journal*, April 1925, 502, 512.
12 *Canada Farmer*, 1 January 1868, 11; *Farmer's Advocate*, February 1869, 25 and April 1869, 55.
13 *Canadian Poultry Chronicle*, July 1870, 3.
14 Ibid.
15 *Canada Farmer*, 15 May 1868, 151.
16 T.F. McGrew, "American Breeds of Poultry," in US Department of Agriculture, Bureau of Animal Industry, *Report*, 1901, 520, 532; *Canadian Poultry Review*, December 1877, 2; *American Poultry Journal*, November 1912, 1539–40; December 1912, 1693, 1696; E. Brown, *Poultry Breeding and Production*, vol. 1 (London: Ernest Benn, 1929), 290–7; O.A. Hanke, ed.,

American Poultry History, 1823–1973 (Madison, WI: American Poultry History Society, 1974), 34–8; E. Brown, *Races of Domestic Poultry*, 150–2.

17 *American Poultry Journal*, January 1907, 33–4.

18 Ibid., 33.

19 *American Poultry Journal*, December 1924, 1119, 1168, 1170–1.

20 Quoted in *Farmer's Advocate*, June 1888, 178.

21 *Canadian Poultry Review*, June 1892, 86.

22 *Farmer's Advocate*, 1 March 1900, 128 and 15 March 1900, 160.

23 *Canadian Poultry Review*, January 1894, 22–3.

24 See, for example, *American Poultry Journal*, August 1925, 756.

25 An interesting discussion of the effects of shows on livestock breeding can be found in E.A. Heaman, *The Inglorious Acts of Peace: Exhibitions in Canadian Society during the Nineteenth Century* (Toronto: University of Toronto Press, 1999).

26 *Canadian Poultry Chronicle*, December 1870, 82.

27 Hanke, ed., *American Poultry History*, 107.

28 *Farmer's Advocate*, 27 October 1927, 1561.

29 See *American Poultry Journal*, August 1922, 806; January 1925, 19, 77, 78–81.

30 Ibid., May 1923, 543.

31 For the linkage in Britain of beefing to purebred genetics, see A. Fraser, *Animal Husbandry Heresies* (London: Crosby Lockwood & Son, 1960), 22–3.

32 Ontario, Department of Agriculture, *Crop Bulletin* no. 3 (August 1882): 18, 20, 22, RG 49, Ontario Department of Agriculture, Statistics and Publications Branch. Triple purpose means cattle that were bred to perform three uses: draft power, beef, and dairy production.

33 Professor William Brown of the Ontario Agricultural College commented on this pattern to the Ontario Agricultural Commission committee in 1880. Ontario Agricultural Commission, *Report*, 1881, vol. 1, 266.

34 *Farmer's Advocate*, July 1887, 194. See also "Our Native Cows," ibid., October, 1881, 247.

35 For more detail on this subject see M. Derry, *Ontario's Cattle Kingdom: Purebred Breeders and Their World, 1870–1920* (Toronto: University of Toronto Press, 2001) and her "The Role of Purebred Breeder/Ordinary Farmer Conflict in the Rate of Herd Improvement – A Study of Cattle Farming in Ontario, 1870–1920," *Proceedings* for the Association of Living Historical Farms and Agricultural Museums Conference, 1998.

36 See good examples of the confusion between purebred genetics and specialization as agents for "improvement" in *Farmer's Advocate*, December 1886, 364; February 1887, 44; July 1887, 194; November 1890, 358; 18 March 1909, 431; *Canadian Breeder and Agricultural Review*, 2

January 1885, 19–20; 8 April 1885, 214; 17 December 1885, 771; *Canadian Live Stock and Farm Journal*, March 1887, 436. For examples of these various confused thoughts on how to breed for purpose, see the following. *Farmer's Advocate*, February 1876, 27; July 1880, 157; October 1883, 299; June 1884, 162; September 1884, 270; June 1886, 170; December 1886, 364; February 1887, 44; July 1887, 194; August 1888, 237; 15 February 1900, 90; 18 March 1909, 431; 29 April 1909, 709–10. Ontario Agricultural Commission, *Report*, 1881, vol. 1, 245, 247, 262, 263, 266, 275; *Farming World and Canadian Farm and Home*, 1 September 1906, 583–4; *Canadian Dairyman and Farming World*, 12 February 1908, 11; *Farm and Dairy and Rural Home*, 15 February 1912, 4, 22; *O.A.C. Review*, October 1891, 3, "A Word about Beefing"; October 1902, 7. For confusion over beef/dairy, see Sessional Paper 3, Legislature of Ontario (henceforth SP, Ontario), 1881, 447–52; SP 23, Ontario, 1884, 53, 97–9. For confusion in *Farmer's Advocate*, see July 1880, 157. For more on various ambiguous recommendations see ibid., September 1884, 270; July 1887, 194; November 1887, 331; August 1888, 237; April 1889, 111–12; April 1890, 109; May 1890, 141; August 1890, 239; September 1890, 279; 15 April 1899, 204; 24 September 1908, 1474; 18 March 1909, 431; 6 October 1910, 1292–3; 2 February 1911, 176; 6 July 1911, 1133. Many breeders continued to breed for single purpose after 1890. See, for example, Sessional Paper 15b, Parliament of Canada (henceforth SP, Canada), 1913, 356–7; *Farming World*, 12 February 1901, 550. For the persistence of dual-purpose thinking, see, for example, *O.A.C. Review*, May 1914, 408. For an imaginative dual-purpose strategy, see *Farm and Dairy & Rural Home*, 13 January 1913, 4.

37 For farmers' views on single purpose, see, for example, *Crop Bulletin*, November 1886, 34–5, November 1899, 9, RG 49, Ontario Department of Agriculture, and "Milk and Beef Together," *Farmer's Advocate*, June 1879, 126.

38 SP 5, Ontario, 1869, 143.

39 Ontario Agricultural Commission, *Report*, 1881, vol. 4, Appendix J, 33.

40 Ibid., vol. 1, 410.

41 Ibid., vol. 4, Appendix G, 52.

42 *Farmer's Advocate*, April 1883, 103.

43 Ibid., 102. See also *Farming*, 16 August, 1898, 429.

44 *Farmer's Advocate*, April 1890, 109; May 1890, 141.

45 SP 3, Ontario, 1882, 111. "Report of the Judges on Prize Farms, 1880."

46 See SP 5, Ontario, 1869, 143, for example.

47 J. Horner, "Changing Spatial Patterns in the Production and Utilization of Milk in Southern Ontario, 1910–1961," MA thesis, University of Toronto, 1967, 34, 61–2, 73. See comparative returns for December 1923

and December 1924 in the *Crop Bulletins* (nos. 157 and 163), RG 49, Public Archives of Ontario.

48 SP 15, Canada, 1914, 46.

49 SP 26, Ontario, 1897, 53.

50 *Farmer's Advocate,* 1 February 1900, 64; 6 May 1909, 753.

51 R. Ankli, "Ontario's Dairy Industry, 1880–1920," *Canadian Papers in Rural History* 8 (1992): 269.

52 For information on milk-testing systems in different countries, see *Publications of the International Institute,* November 1912, 31–41; *Canadian Live-Stock and Farm Journal,* August 1885, 212. *Farmer's Advocate* stated in 1892 that the average cow in Ontario yielded 3,000 lbs. a year; January 1892, 21. In 1895 the journal implied that a cow should give 5,000 lbs. a year in order to be profitable; 15 October 1895, 415; Ankli, "Ontario's Dairy Industry," 268–70. See also Committee on Agricultural Conditions, Dominion Government of Canada, *Report,* 1924, Part 2, 461–75; *Farmer's Advocate,* 27 July 1916, 1252, for an example of the production of purebred cattle. A. Leitch, "Farm Management, 1919, Part II. The Beef Raising Business in Western Ontario, the Mixed Farming Business in Western Ontario, the Dairying Farming Business in Eastern Ontario," Bulletin 278, Ontario Agricultural College, Ontario Department of Agriculture, June 1920, 11, 13.

53 See Canada, Parliament, *Proceedings* of the Special Committee on the Cost of Living, 1919, 181, 190, 201 for information on labour and both beef and dairy production. For the labour shortage, see *Farmer's Advocate,* 6 May 1916, 787; 16 May 1916, 878c; 7 January 1915, 10; 1 June 1916, 957; 5 April 1917, 572. See also *O.A.C Review,* September 1917, 6 and April 1916, 304. Note also that in 1913 Holstein transfers were only two-thirds that of Shorthorn transfers, while by 1920 Holstein transfers exceeded those of Shorthorns. *Farmer's Advocate,* 20 February 1920, 258. *Twentieth Century Impressions of Canada,* ed. H. Boam (Montreal: Sells, 1914), 251. *Farmer's Advocate,* 20 February 1920, 258.

54 For more on calf killing and ethical issues, see M. Derry, *Masterminding Nature: The Breeding of Animals, 1750–2010* (Toronto: University of Toronto Press, 2015), chapter 6.

55 See L.T.G. Theunissen, *Beauty or Statistics: Practice and Science in Dutch Livestock Breeding 1900–2000* (Toronto: University of Toronto Press, 2020), chapter 1; his "Breeding without Mendelism: Theory and Practice of Dairy Cattle Breeding in the Netherlands, 1900–1950," *Journal of the History of Biology* 41 (2008): 637–76; and his "Breeding for Nobility or Production? Cultures of Dairy Cattle Breeding in the Netherlands, 1945–1995," *Isis* 103 (2012): 278–309.

56 G. Adami, "On the Significance of Bovine Tuberculosis and Its Eradication and Prevention in Canada," a paper given at the Canadian Medical Association in 1899 and printed in SP 14, Ontario, 1902.
57 SP 15b, Canada, 1913, 336. As a young man, Rutherford actually worked as a veterinarian at Bow Park. See also L. Cox, '"Reasonable Tact and Diplomacy': Disease Management and Bovine Tuberculosis in North America, 1890–1950," PhD thesis, University of Guelph, 2013, 142. See also Derry, *Ontario's Cattle Kingdom*, 65–71.
58 Cox, '"Reasonable Tact and Diplomacy,'" 14, 109, 114, 117.
59 For more on this subject, see M. Derry, *Horses in Society: A Story of Breeding and Marketing Culture, 1800–1920* (Toronto: University of Toronto Press, 2006) and her "The Transition from Type to Breed: Draft Horses and Purebred Breeding in the International American Market, 1870–1920," in *Horse Breeds and Human Society: Purity, Identity and the Making of the Modern Horse*, ed. Kristen Guest and Monica Hattfeld (London: Routledge Press, 2020).
60 Ontario Agricultural Commission, *Report*, 1881, vol. 1, 434–5.
61 *Breeder's Gazette*, 23 February 1882, 311.
62 *Farmer's Advocate*, 1 November 1905, 809.
63 Ibid., 25 September 1913, 1672.
64 Ibid., January 1883, 5.
65 *Farming World for Stockmen and Farmers*, 22 April 1902, 415–21.
66 *Farmer's Advocate*, May 1887, 133.
67 Ibid., November 1884, 334.
68 Ibid., February 1878, 41.
69 *Breeder's Gazette*, 27 April 1882, 565; 31 August 1882, 301.
70 Ibid., 27 January 1892, 72–3.
71 Ibid., 16 March 1892, 211.
72 Ibid., 17 July 1895, 43.
73 Ibid., 29 January 1896, 74.
74 Ibid., 26 February 1896, 153.
75 Ibid., 26 August 1896, 137.
76 *Farming World and Canadian Farm and Home*, 1 June 1904, 421.
77 *Farmer's Advocate*, 15 March 1906, 398–9.
78 Ibid., 1 May 1913, 814.
79 Ibid., 30 January 1913, 168.
80 Ibid., 18 July 1912, 1278.
81 *Breeder's Gazette*, 15 April 1891, 299.
82 *Farmer's Advocate*, 29 April 1915, 713.
83 Belgians had made inroads in the heavy horse world by this time. They competed with Percherons, because Belgians lacked the hairy legs of the Clyde.

5. Implications of Breeding for Colour

1 M. Derry, *Art and Science in Breeding: Creating Better Chickens* (Toronto: University of Toronto Press, 2012), 45–54.
2 *Farmer's Advocate*, 14 December 1916, 2046.
3 See, for example, *American Poultry Journal*, May 1911, 1006.
4 T.F. McGrew, "American Breeds of Poultry," in US Department of Agriculture, Bureau of Animal Industry, *Report*, 1901, 525, 531–2; *American Poultry Journal*, March 1909, 307; August 1913, 1135–7; October 1923, 989, 1015.
5 See *The Plymouth Rocks, Barred, White and Buff* (Quincy, IL: Reliable Poultry Journal Publishing Company, 1899), 23–6; *American Poultry Journal*, April 1907, 365–6; April 1908, 330–1.
6 *American Poultry Journal*, April 1915, 676.
7 *The Plymouth Rocks*, 26; *American Poultry Journal*, January 1922, 56, 58.
8 *The Plymouth Rocks*, 31.
9 *American Poultry Journal*, October 1915, 1229, 1243; November 1915, 1315–16.
10 G. MacEwan, *Highlights of Shorthorn History* (Winnipeg: Hignell Printing, 1982), 78 and quoted from John Clay, manager of the company that owned Bow Park, *My Recollections of Ontario* (Chicago: Private Printing, 1918), 56, 79.
11 Sessional Paper 6, Legislature of Ontario (henceforth SP, Ontario), 1878, 11.
12 "The Red, White and Roan – Which Color Should We Adopt?" *Canadian Live-Stock and Farm Journal*, July 1886, 176. See also "Colour versus Quality in Shorthorns," *O.A.C. Review*, May 1896, 2.
13 *Farmer's Advocate*, 11 March 1909, 380–1.
14 Johnston to a breeder in Quebec, 27 May 1902, Letterbook 7, Johnston Papers, Public Archives of Ontario.
15 SP 20, Ontario, 1895, 47.
16 *Canadian Live-Stock and Farm Journal*, September 1885, 226; July 1886, 176.
17 Ibid., March 1885, 59.
18 Johnston to J. Watters, 14, 20 September 1901, Letterbook 6, Johnston Papers.
19 Cruickshank to James Davidson, 8 January 1882, 17 June 1887, Miller-Davidson Papers, University of Guelph Archives.
20 *Breeder's Gazette*, 1 December 1881, 7.
21 Ibid., 29 December 1881, 102.
22 Ibid., 15 December 1881, 51.
23 A. Sanders, *Short-Horn Cattle, a Series of Historical Sketches, Memoirs and Records of the Breed and Its Development in the United States and Canada* (Chicago: Sanders Publishing, 1900), 854–5.

24 A. Sanders, *Red, White and Roan* (Chicago: American Shorthorn Breeders' Association, 1936), 619.
25 *O.A.C. Review*, October 1904, 13.
26 Great Britain, *Journal of the Ministry of Agriculture* 28 (May 1921): 110–11; A. Fraser, *Animal Husbandry Heresies* (London: Crosby Lockwood & Son, 1960), 64–6.
27 For a rather good discussion of roaning patterns, and illustrations of them, see B.K. Green, *The Color of Horses* (Northland Press, 1974), 103–9.
28 C.F. McClary, "Opening Remarks," Ninth Annual Session, National Poultry Breeders' Roundtable, 1960, 2; A.W. Nordskog, "The Evolution of Animal Breeding Practices – Commercial and Experimental," Fourteenth Annual Session, National Poultry Breeders' Roundtable, 1965, 58–9, 72.
29 E. Brown, *Races of Domestic Poultry* (London: Edward Arnold, 1906), 72, 73, 60–7; O.A. Hanke, ed., *American Poultry History, 1823–1973* (Madison, WI: American Poultry History Society, 1974), 34–8.
30 D.K. Flock and R. Preisinger, "Specialization and Concentration as Contributing Factors to the Success of the Poultry Industry in the Global Food Market," draft, *Lohmann Information* (Winter 2007): 4.
31 *Poultry Tribune*, August 1985.
32 The single word "Collie" is attached to only one breed of dog, even though a number of sheep dog breeds are considered to be "collie" types. See M. Derry, *Bred for Perfection: Shorthorn Cattle, Collies, and Arabian Horses since 1800* (Baltimore: Johns Hopkins University Press, 2003), 68, for a chart describing the relationship of different collie-type breeds to each other, particularly the connections between the Border Collie, the Shetland Sheepdog, and the Collie. Early in the twentieth century, Shetland Sheepdog breeders campaigned for the right to call their dogs "collies" and lost. See ibid., 93–4, for that story. The breed, known simply as the Collie, comes in two versions, rough and smooth. The versions are divided only by the length of coat.
33 For more on white Collies, see M. Derry, "White Collies, Beauty or Genetic Defect: Regulation and Breeding, 1870–2013," *Society and Animals* 28 (2020): 472–88.
34 O.P. Bennett and T.M. Halpin, *The Collie* (Washington, IL: O.P. Bennett, 1942), 21.
35 Quoted in *Canadian Poultry Review*, December 1877, 103.
36 M. Devine, *Border Collies* (New York: Barron's, 1997), 10.
37 Contemporary painted images of these white dogs provide strong evidence that they resulted from merle to merle breeding.
38 *Collie Folio*, October 1909, 351; E.C. Ash, *Dogs: Their History and Development*, vol. 1 (London: Ernest Benn, 1927), 278.
39 See K. White, "Victorian and Edwardian Dogs," *Veterinary History* ns 7 (1992): 72–7.

40 *Collie Folio*, October 1909, 351; Ash, *Dogs*, vol. 1, 278.
41 *Country Life in America*, November 1915, np.
42 K. Marshall, *His Dogs: Albert Payson Terhune and the Sunnybank Collies* (New York: Collie Club of America Foundation [Collie Health Foundation], 2001), 64.
43 L. Rorem, "White Collies," http://izebug.syr.edu/~gsbisco/white/whitec.htm, accessed 30 July 1999.
44 G. Kaye, *The Collie in America* (Valley Center, CA: Chelsea, 2008), 385.
45 Giulia Faessler and Lucio Rocco, "History of the White Collie," http://www.pastorescozzese.com/storia/bianco_e.htm, accessed 12 November 2014; Kaye, *The Collie in America*, 387.
46 Ibid., 385.
47 Ibid., 386.
48 *Collie Folio*, September 1910, 313.
49 Faessler and Rocco, "History of the White Collie."
50 G. Gaye, "A Century of Collies and Significant Developments: Part IV," *Collie Expressions* (April–May 2000): 51.
51 Faessler and Rocco, "History of the White Collie."
52 Kaye, *The Collie in America*, 389.
53 Standard Review Committee, Collie Club of America, *Report*, 2009, 16.
54 A.L. Mitchell, "Dominant Dilution and Other Color Factors in Collie Dogs," *Journal of Heredity* 26 (1935): 425–30. See also R.M. Kleinman, "The Inheritance of Coat Color in the American Collie," MSc thesis, Western Reserve University, 1949.
55 C.C. Little, *The Inheritance of Coat Color in Dogs* (New York: Howell, 1971; 1st ed. Ithaca: Comstock Pub. Associates, 1957).
56 Colour genetics in dogs is complicated and can vary by breed. Many books deal with the subject, from a scientist's and a breeder's point of view. See in particular Little, *The Inheritance of Coat Color in Dogs*.
57 See G.M. Strain et al., "Prevalence of Deafness in Dogs Heterozygous or Homozygous for the Merle Allele," *Journal of Veterinary Internal Medicine* 23 (2009): 282–6.
58 L.A. Clark et al., "Retrotransposon Insertion of *SILV* Is Responsible for Merle Patterning in the Domestic Dog," *Proceedings of the National Academy of Sciences* 103 (2006): 1376–81.
59 See the websites for Rainshade Collies, Wyndlair Collies, and Deep River Collies. An ad for a show double merle can be seen in *Collie Cues*, July/August 1985, 19.
60 See, for example, "White Collies? Have You Heard of Them? Any Health Problems?" http://www.dogforums.com/general-dog-forum/109173-white-collies-h, accessed 26 January 2014.
61 "Westminster Dog Show. Do They Really Care?" http://answers.yahoo.com/question/index?qid=20120213160532AAjkxaE, accessed 25 January 2014.

62 Marianne Sullivan, "Merle to Merle Breeding," *AKC Gazette* 29 (March 2012): 34.
63 Ibid., 35.
64 S.L. Vanderlip, *The Collie: A Veterinary Reference for the Professional Breeder* (Cardiff by the Sea, CA: Biotechnical Veterinary Consultants, 1984), 44.
65 Faessler and Rocco, "History of the White Collie."
66 "European Convention for the Protection of Pet Animals," European Treaty Series no. 125, Strasbourg, 13 November 1987. http://conventions.coe.int/Treaty/Commun/QueVoulezVous.asp?CL=ENG&NT=125; http://conventions.coe.int/Treaty/en/Treaties/Html/125.htm, accessed 24 September 2014.
67 http://www.fci.be/en/Breeding-42.html, accessed 10 December 2015.
68 J. Turner, *Animal Breeding, Welfare and Society* (London: Routledge; New York: Earthscan, 2010), 128, 146–7.
69 http://www.thekennelclub.org.uk/services/public/breed/restrictions.aspx?id=6151, accessed 12 April 2014.

6. Breeding for Authenticity

1 R. Nash, "A Perfect Nicking Pattern," *Humanimalia* 10 (2018): 37–9.
2 *Tesio: In His Own Words*, trans. M. Burnett (Neenah, WI: Russell Meerdink, 2005). The original version, F. Tesio's *Puro-Sangue – Animale da Experimento*, was published in 1947 in Milan. Tesio adds an almost religious element to his breeding theories, as well as the presence of love in any act of reproduction. The results of his horse-breeding operations proved to be spectacular.
3 For more on this subject, see M. Derry, *Bred for Perfection: Shorthorn Cattle, Collies, and Arabian Horses since 1800* (Baltimore: Johns Hopkins University Press, 2003).
4 O. Barnum, "Who Is Breeding the Old-Fashioned Collie?" *Country Life in America*, 15 December 1911, np.
5 R.A. Sturdevant, "The Case for the Modern Collie," ibid., 1 March 1912, np.
6 "Save the Old-Fashioned Collie!" ibid., 15 March 1912, np.
7 "The Old-Fashioned Collie," ibid., 15 August 1912, np.
8 *Collie Folio*, 12 May 1912, 167.
9 Robert Preston to J.P. Morgan Jr, 13 August 1918, Box 105, J.P. Morgan Jr Papers, Pierpont Morgan Library Archives, New York.
10 J.P. Morgan Jr's secretary to R. Preston, 18 August 1918, ibid.
11 "Friends of the Old Farm Collie, Bulletin 1," February 1995, http://izebug.syr.edu/~gsbisco/bull1a.htm, accessed 30 July 1999.

12 "Classic Victorian Collie Club," http://izebug.syr.edu/~gsbisco/bull5b.htm, accessed 29 July 1999.
13 American Working Farmcollie Association, http://www.geocities.com/farmcollie1, accessed 8 February 2001.
14 http://www.farmcollie.com/mission-statement.htm, accessed 4 June 2019.
15 See http://www.farmcollie.com/, accessed 4 June 2019.
16 For more on this subject, see Derry, *Bred for Perfection*.
17 A few examples are H.H. Reese, *The Kellogg Arabians: Their Background and Influence* (Alhambra, CA: Bordon Publishing Company, 1958), 27, 30, 34; J. Forbis, *The Classic Arabian Horse* (New York: Liveright, 1976), 254–5, 276; "Davenport Arabians at Craver Farms," *Arabiana*, 10–11; G.B. Edwards-Craver letters, ibid., 15, 98–9; D.S. Whitman, "The Strain of It All," *American Arabian Online*, http://www.geocities.com/Heartland/Ranch/7485/strain.html, accessed 28 August 1999; Lady Wentworth, *The Authentic Arabian Horse* (London: George Allen and Urwin, 1945; 3rd ed. 1979), 143, 314; G.B. Edwards, "To Progress ... or Regress That Is the Question," *Arab Horse Journal* (henceforth *AHJ*), May 1960, 12–16; G.B. Edwards, "The Great Strain Robbery or Pursuit of the Pashas," Part 1, *AHJ*, August 1960, 22–4, 29; G.B. Edwards, "The Great Strain Robbery or Pursuit of the Pashas," Part 2, *AHJ*, September 1960, 22–6, 28; "Arabian Horses," *Canadian Breeder and Agricultural Review*, 8 April 1885, 214; E.B. Babcock and R.E. Clausen, *Genetics in Relation to Agriculture* (New York: McGraw-Hill Book Company, 1918), 444; E. Skorkowski, "Three Arabian Races," *AHJ*, June 1960, 30–2.
18 Wentworth, *The Authentic Arabian Horse*, 89–91.
19 Edwards, "To Progress," 13–14.
20 Mohammed Ali and Abbas Pasha, *Arabian Horse World* (henceforth *AHW*), May 1982, 336–8, 343. Both the May 1981 and the May 1982 editions of the *AHW* have many articles on the history of the Arabian horse in relation to Egypt. See also the Preface and "Historic Sketch of the Rise and Decline of Wahhabism in Arabia" by Wilfrid Blunt in Lady Anne Blunt, *A Pilgrimage to Nejd* (1881; reprint London: Century Publishing Co., 1985).
21 See Forbis, *The Classic Arabian Horse*. She sets Egypt, not Arabia, as the acknowledged centre, and therefore the font of Arabian horse breeding.
22 K. Ott, "Blue Star Arabians, Blue List Arabians, and Arabians," *Arabiana*, 133.
23 J.L. Ott, "Arabian Types and Strains, 'Egyptian', 'Blunt' and 'Crabbet,'" ibid., 152.
24 Quoted in Forbis, *The Classic Arabian Horse*, 135.

25 See S. Swart and G. Bankoff, eds., *Breeds of Empire: The "Invention" of the Horse in Southeast Asia and Southern Africa* (Copenhagen: Nordic Institute of Asian Studies Press, 2007).
26 Ali Pasha Sherif, *AHW*, May 1982, 343–4.
27 M. Greely, *Arabian Exodus* (London: J.A. Allen, 1975), 30–5; Reese, *The Kellogg Arabians*, 39–40; Forbis, *The Classic Arabian Horse*, 159; G.B. Edwards, "The Great Strain Robbery or the Pursuit of the Pashas," Part 2, 12–13; G.B. Edwards, "Glass Eyes and White Markings in Arabs," *AHJ*, April 1959, 20; M. Weise, "A Reference Guide: Arabian Color Coat," http://www.arabian-horses.com/feature/margo/color/, accessed 16 September 1999; J. Forbis, "The Arabian Horse in the Middle East," Part 3, *AHJ*, July 1960, 22.
28 Greely, *Arabian Exodus*, 44.
29 Reese, *The Kellogg Arabians*, 43.
30 Wentworth's book, *The Authentic Arabian Horse*, provides a detailed description of her views on breeding, strains, and authenticity in the true Arabian.
31 Forbis, *The Classic Arabian Horse*, 254, 275.
32 "Raswan," *Arabiana*, 148; J.L. Ott, "Arabian Types and Strains,'" 142, 145, 152; "Davenport Arabians at Craver Farms," 10–11; G.B. Edwards, letter, *Arabiana*, 15.
33 Reese, *The Kellogg Arabians*, 101.
34 J.L. Ott, "Arabian Types and Strains,'" 142, 145, 152; K. Ott, "Blue Star Arabians," 142, 145, 152.
35 "Davenport Arabians at Craver Farms," 3, 6, 11, 98, 141.
36 K. Ott, "Blue Star Arabians," 133.
37 Reese, *The Kellogg Arabians*, 35.
38 G.B. Edwards, letter, *Arabiana*, 15.
39 Edwards, "To Progress," 12–16.
40 Kellogg to Wentworth, 3 November 1926, W.K. Kellogg Arabian Horse Library, W.K. Kellogg Arabian Horse Ranch Records 0019, Series 1: Correspondence "W" Miscellaneous 1927 – "X" "Y" "Z" Miscellaneous 1927 (Wentworth, Lady), Box 40, Special Collections and Archives, Cal Poly Ponoma University Library.
41 Kellogg to Wentworth, 10 April 1926, ibid.
42 Kellogg to Wentworth, 8 June 1926, ibid.
43 Kellogg to Wentworth, 28 June 1926, ibid.
44 Wentworth to Captain Milbanke, 8 August 1926, ibid.
45 Wentworth to Kellogg, 24 August 1926, ibid.
46 Brown wrote a book about his adventures in Arabia and about his theories concerning the breeding of the Arabian horse. In it he makes no

reference to Raswan. See W.R. Brown, *The Horse of the Desert* (New York: Macmillan Company, 1929, reprint 1947).

47 W.R. Brown to W.K. Kellogg, 8 June 1929, W.K. Kellogg Arabian Horse Library.

48 E. Russell, for example, in his *Greyhound Nation: A Coevolutionary History of England, 1200–1900* (Cambridge: Cambridge University Press, 2018), describes improvement breeding as selective breeding as a way to differentiate the two.

49 J.L. Ott, "Arabian Types and Strains,'" 146.

50 Forbis, *The Classic Arabian Horse*, 416.

51 See M. Worboys, J.-M. Strange, and N. Pemberton, *The Invention of the Modern Dog: Breed and Blood in Victorian Britain* (Baltimore: Johns Hopkins University Press, 2018).

7. Pedigree versus No Pedigree and the Market Value of Animals

1 See, for example, J. Walton, "The Diffusion of Improved Shorthorn Cattle in Britain During the Eighteenth and Nineteenth Centuries," *Transactions of the Institute of British Geographers* ns 9 (1984): 22–36, and his "Pedigree and the National Cattle Herd circa 1750–1950," *Agricultural History Review* 34 (1986): 149–70; E. Whetham, "The Trade in Pedigree Livestock, 1850–1910," ibid., 27 (1979): 47–50.

2 A. Sanders, *Short-Horn Cattle, a Series of Historical Sketches, Memoirs and Records of the Breed and Its Development in the United States and Canada* (Chicago: Sanders Publishing, 1900), 199–202.

3 C.B. Plumb, "Felix Renick, Pioneer," *Ohio Archaeological and Historical Publications* 38 (1924): 21–2, 28–30, 35–41; P. Henlein, "Cattle Kingdom in the Ohio Valley: The Beef Cattle Industry in the Ohio Valley, 1783–1860," PhD thesis, University of Wisconsin, 1957, 93; Sanders, *Short-Horn Cattle*, 199–202.

4 Plumb, "Felix Renick, Pioneer," 35–50.

5 See S. Wright, "Mendelian Analysis of the Pure Bred Breeds of Livestock, Part 1: The Measurement of Inbreeding and Relationship," *Journal of Heredity* 14 (1923): 339–48, and "Mendelian Analysis of the Pure Breeds of Livestock. Part 2: The Duchess Family of Shorthorns As Bred by Thomas Bates," ibid., 405–22.

6 G. MacEwan, *Highlights of Shorthorn History* (Winnipeg: Hignill Printing, 1982), 36, 70.

7 D. Marshall, *Shorthorn Cattle in Canada* (Dominion Shorthorn Association, 1932), 117–26, 211.

8 Sanders, *Short-Horn Cattle*, 450.

9 *Farmer's Advocate*, 30 September 1873, cited in Marshall, *Shorthorn Cattle in Canada*, 240.
10 Sanders, *Short-Horn Cattle*, 510, 712–13, 720.
11 Sessional Paper 26, Legislature of Ontario (henceforth SP, Ontario), 1897, 127.
12 It should be noted in passing that pedigree/tariff problems affected the international trade in purebred light horses as well. In 1910, for example, Canadian and American breeders of Hackney horses became reluctant to import from Britain, because "a large percentage of those imported last year would not record in Canada" or the United States. Americans and Canadians jointly tried to make British breeders modify standards to bring them more in line with North American ones, but apparently made little progress. See *Farmer's Advocate*, 29 December 1910, 2075.
13 See, for example, *Breeder's Gazette*, 17 December 1902, 1232; 14 February 1900, 203–4; 25 March 1891, 237; 24 January 1900, 108; 21 February 1900, 234; 5 August 1903, 207.
14 *Accounts and Papers [4]: Army (Militia), Army and Volenteers* (1902); *Proceedings of a Court of enquiry on the Administration of the Army Remount since 1899* (1902); *Horse Breeding: Bills to Regulate the Use of Stallions for Stud Purposes* (1918); *Minutes of Evidence Taken before the Departmental Committee to Appointed to Enquire and Report as the British Trade in Live Stock with the Colonies and Other Countries* (1912), Cd. 6032; *Report from the Select Committee of the House of Lords on Horses; Together with the proceedings of the Committee, Minutes of Evidence, and Appendix* (1873); *Reports of the Royal Commission on Horse Breeding* (1888–1911), of which the 1890 report is the most important.
15 See M.E. Derry, *Bred for Perfection: Shorthorn Cattle, Collies, and Arabian Horses since 1800* (Baltimore: Johns Hopkins University Press, 2003), 1–16; *Horses in Society: A Story of Breeding and Marketing Culture, 1800–1920* (Toronto: University of Toronto Press, 2006), 3–25; *Masterminding Nature: The Breeding of Animals, 1750–2010* (Toronto: University of Toronto Press, 2015), 13–39.
16 United Kingdom, *Third Report of the Royal Commission on Horse Breeding*, 1890, 3, 4, 46–7, 89–91, 109, 111.
17 Ibid., 8.
18 Ibid., 19, 35.
19 For a more thorough discussion of the 1890 report of the British Horse Commission, see Derry, *Horses in Society*, 159–71.
20 State encouragement, rather than legislative action, promoted the use of purebred cattle, pig, and sheep males in the same period. The movement never had the teeth that stallion legislation had. Encouragement rather than force, for example, dominated cattle

improvement activities in the United States and Canada. An American campaign against "scrub" bulls was initially triggered by concerns over the quality of beef cattle in relation to stock being raised in Argentina. "Better Bulls," Bulletin 281, Ontario Agricultural College, Ontario Department of Agriculture, 1920, 5. American farmers were encouraged to use purebred bulls through a number of financial incentives. Cooperative bull associations, in which farmers owned a bull jointly, also developed, with the first being established in 1906 in Michigan. H.A. Herman, *Improving Cattle by the Millions: NAAB and the Development and Worldwide Application of Artificial Insemination* (Columbia: University of Missouri Press, 1981), 7, 8. In Canada, a system of loaning purebred bulls to farmers' associations across the country was in place by 1909. Sessional Paper 15a, Parliament of Canada (henceforth SP, Canada), 1909, 48. No legislation was advocated (or indeed put in place) to force farmers to abandon their non-purebred bulls. Increased federal government financial support came in the form of the Sire Loaning Policy and Sire Purchasing Policy, both designed to help farmers buy purebred superior bulls more cheaply. SP 15, Canada, 1920, 21; SP 15, Canada, 1923, 72.

21 C.C. Glenn, "Stallion Legislation and the Horse-Breeding Industry," *Yearbook*, US, Department of Agriculture, 1916, 290, 296. *Breeder's Gazette*, 2 March 1916, 495. For a more thorough discussion about stallion enrolment in the United States, see Derry, *Horses in Society*, 172–201; *Farmer's Advocate*, 1 August 1918, 1265; 18 July 1912, 1279; *Farm and Dairy*, 15 August 1918, 887; *Agricultural Gazette* of Canada 7 (1920): 413, 490; ibid. 1 (1914): 187; ibid. 6 (1919): 1057.

22 *Breeder's Gazette*, 23 May 1888, 521–2.

23 Ibid., 30 May 1888, 546–7; 6 June 1888, 572.

24 See *Farming World and Canadian Farm and Home*, 1 February 1906, np; 15 March 1904, 213; 15 March 1907, 254; *Farming World for Farmers and Stockmen*, 1 April 1903, 39; 1 April 1903, 158; *Farmer's Advocate*, 4 October 1906, 1556. Saskatchewan Department of Agriculture, *Report*, 1919, 240; SP 15b, Canada, 1913, 381.

25 *Canadian Dairyman and Farming World*, 19 February 1908, 12; *Farmer's Advocate* (Western version), 9 March 1910, 1595; SP 15b, Canada, 1913, 381–2; *Farmer's Advocate*, 15 March 1901, 187.

26 *Farming World and Canadian Farm and Home*, 15 June 1905, 453; Glenn, "Stallion Legislation and the Horse-Breeding Industry," 289–90.

27 *Farming World and Canadian Farm and Home*, 1 February 1907, 99, 100.

28 R.A. Cave, "State Legislation Regulating the Standing of Stallions and Jacks for Public Service," US Department of Agriculture, Bureau of Animal Industry, *Report*, 1908, 336.

29 See, for example, *Breeder's Gazette*, 11 April, 1906, 788; 30 March 1910, 811; 4 January 1911, 23; 18 January 1911, 148; 1 February 1911, 280; 8 February 1911, 352; 13 February 1913, 596; 12 April 1911, 946; 19 April 1911, 1004.
30 For example, in the United States, see *Breeder's Gazette*, 30 May 1888, 546–7; 23 March 1904, 566–7; 20 December 1905, 1309; 17 June 1903, 1173; 12 April 1911, 946. For Canada, see SP 22, Ontario, 1909, 180–4; SP 65, Ontario, 1907, "Special Investigation on Horse Breeding in Ontario, 1906."
31 For example, in 1921, at the end of the period under discussion in relation to stallion regulation in the province of Ontario (which is focused on here), purebred cattle numbered fifty-five to every thousand head of cattle. *Census* of Canada, 1921, vol. 5, xc, 64. See as well the pamphlet "Better Bulls," released by the Ontario Department of Agriculture in 1920, and the exhaustive 1936 report of the USDA on animal and plant breeding, *Better Plants and Animals*.
32 SP 23, Ontario, 1900, 15.
33 *Farmer's Advocate*, 27 April, 1905, 623.
34 Ibid., 29 March 1906, 493; SP 39, Ontario, 1914, 65.
35 See SP 65, Ontario, 1907, "Special Investigation on Horse Breeding in Ontario, 1906," 12, 15.
36 See, for example, ibid., 18, 20, 24, 31, 33.
37 Ibid., 20, 23, 36, 39.
38 *Canadian Dairyman and Farming World*, 19 February 1908, 12.
39 *Farming World and Canadian Farm and Home*, 15 November 1906, 789. See as well SP 65, Ontario, 1907 for "Special Investigation on Horse Breeding in Ontario, 1906."
40 *Farming World and Canadian Farm and Home*, 15 November 1906, 789.
41 Ibid., 1 December 1906, 819; *Farmer's Advocate*, 6 December 1906, 1888; 1 November 1906, 1692.
42 *Farmer's Advocate*, 10 January 1907, 43.
43 *Farming World and Canadian Farm and Home*, 15 March 1907, 254.
44 SP 22, Ontario, 1909, 167.
45 SP 39, Ontario, 1914, 65.
46 SP 22, Ontario, 1909, 180–4. This document covers discussions from the meetings which are presented here.
47 Ibid., 170–5.
48 Interview with Dr Ray J. Geor, Ontario Veterinary College, University of Guelph, 11 February 2004.
49 *Farmer's Advocate*, 12 September 1912, 1607.
50 Ibid., 8 January 1914, 43, 50; 22 January 1914, 132; 29 January 1914, 175, 176.
51 Ibid., 8 January 1914, 43, 50.

52 Ibid., 22 January 1914, 132.
53 Ibid., 29 January 1914, 175, 176.
54 "Stallion Enrolment," *Agricultural Gazette* 1 (1914): 221.
55 SP 39, Ontario, 1915, 5.
56 Ibid., 13.
57 *Farmer's Advocate*, 23 April 1914, 811; SP 39, Ontario, 1915, 5; *Breeder's Gazette*, 24 December 1914, 1145.
58 *Farmer's Advocate*, 4 March 1915, 337.
59 Ibid., 2 November 1916, 1799.
60 K. Voth, "From Big to Small to Big to Small: Part 2 of a Pictorial History of Cattle Changes over the Years," *On Pasture*, 11 July 2016, 1–2 (based on the research of Harlan Ritchie of Michigan State University on the history of beef cattle styles), http://onpasture.com/2016/07/11/from-big-to-small-to-big-to-small-part-2-of-a-pictorial-history-of-cattle-changes-over-the-years. accessed 13 July 2016.
61 See, for example, the address given by C.F. Curtiss, director and professor of agriculture at the State Agricultural College and Experimental Farm, Ames, Iowa, to the superintendent of Farmer Institutes of Ontario in 1897; Curtiss, "The Fundamental Points of Practical Excellence in Beef Cattle," SP 23, Ontario, 1897, 80–5. For comments concerning the commonality of vision in the American and Canadian breeding of Shorthorns, see SP 4, Ontario, 1877, 188.
62 Derry, *Ontario's Cattle Kingdom*, 22; *Directories of the Breeders of Pure Bred Stock of the Dominion of Canada, Dairy Branch*, Live Stock Division (Ottawa: Department of Agriculture, 1901–20). In Ontario, for example, there were seventeen purebreds per one thousand head of cattle, and in 1921 there were fifty-five per one thousand. See *Census of Canada 1911*, vol. 4, 410, 418; *Census of Canada 1921*, vol. 5, xc, 64. The situation in the United States was similar, and the purebred industries of both countries were closely linked from at least the 1870s.
63 B.K. Whitlock, L. Kaiser, and H.S. Maxwell, "Heritable Bovine Fetal Abnormalities," *Theriogenology* 70 (August 2008): 539; P.W. Gregory, W.S. Tyler, and L.M. Julian, "Bovine Achondroplasia: The Reconstitution of the Dexter Components from Non-Dexter Stock," *Growth* 30 (1966): 393–418; P.W. Gregory and F.D. Carroll, "Evidence for the Same Dwarf Gene in Hereford, Aberdeen-Angus, and Certain Other Breeds of Cattle," *Journal of Heredity* 47, no. 3 (1956): 110; E.W. Stringam, "Dwarfism in Beef Cattle," *Canadian Journal of Comparative Medicine and Veterinary Science* 22 (1958): 401; M.L. Baker, C.T. Blunn, and M.M. Oloufa, "Stumpy: A Recessive Achondroplasia in Shorthorn Cattle," *Journal of Heredity* 41, no. 9 (1950): 243–5.
64 K.P. Bovard and L.N. Hazel, "Growth Patterns in Snorter Dwarf and Normal Hereford Calves," *Journal of Animal Science* 22, no. 1 (1963): 194.

65 Whitlock, Kaiser, and Maxwell, "Heritable Bovine Fetal Abnormalities," 539; Thomas J. Marlowe, "Evidence of Selection for the Snorter Dwarf Gene in Cattle," *Journal of Animal Science* 23, no. 2 (1964): 454, 459; M.L. Baker, C.T. Blunn, and M. Plum, "'Dwarfism' in Aberdeen-Angus Cattle," *Journal of Heredity* 42, no. 3 (1951): 143; P.W. Gregory et al., "A Phenotypic Expression of Homozygous Dwarfism in Beef Cattle," *Journal of Animal Science* 10, no. 4 (1951): 923; J.I. Sprague, Jr, W.T. Magee, and R.H. Nelson, "A Pedigree Analysis of Aberdeen-Angus Cattle," *Journal of Heredity* 52, no. 3 (1961): 129–32.
66 O.F. Pahnish, E.B. Stanley, and C.E. Safley, "The Inheritance of a Dwarf Anomaly in Beef Cattle," *Journal of Animal Science* 14, no. 1 (1955): 200; L.E. Johnson, G.S. Harshfield, and W. McCone, "Dwarfism: An Hereditary Defect in Beef Cattle," *Journal of Heredity* 41, no. 7 (1950): 177–81.
67 Whitlock, Kaiser, and Maxwell, "Heritable Bovine Fetal Abnormalities," 539.
68 Voth, "From Big to Small to Big to Small: Part 2," 13; Voth, "From Big to Small to Big to Small: Part 3 of a Pictorial History of Cattle Changes over the Years," *On Pasture*, 18 July 2016, 10–11, http://onpasture.com/2016/07/18/from-big-to-small-to-big-to-small-part-3-of-a-pictorial-history-of-cattle-over-the-years/, accessed 18 July 2016.
69 J. Howse, "Champion's Demotion," *Maclean's*, 9 March 1987, 6.
70 H. Witt, "Perfection Turns Out to Be Just a Lot of Bull," *Chicago Tribune*, 29 July 1987, np.
71 Craig Huffhines, "History of Greats," *Hereford World*, December 2012, 6–7.
72 Hereford Talk, "The Perfection Case," 4 December 2012, herefordtalk.com.
73 Ibid.
74 See http://www.usef.org/content/equestrianSports/breeds/nationalShowHorse.php, and http://www.imh.org/imh/bw/natshow.html, accessed 17 November 2004; *Arabian Horse World* (henceforth *AHW*), February 1983, 352.
75 *AHW*, February 1983, 352; April 1983, 406; June 1983, 541; June 1985, 98–9; August 1985, 96–107; September 1985, 333.
76 For more on both standardbred breeding and the Standardbred trotting horse, see Derry, *Horses in Society*, and her *Masterminding Nature*. See also P. Thurtle, "Harnessing Heredity in Gilded Age America: Middle Class Mores and Industrial Breeding in a Cultural Context," *Journal of the History of Biology* 35 (2002): 43–78.
77 See L.T.G. Theunissen, "The Transformation of the Dutch Farm Horse into a Riding Horse: Livestock Breeding, Science, and Modernization, 1960s–1980s," *Agricultural History* 92 (2018): 24–53; and his *Beauty or*

Statistics: Practice and Science in Dutch Livestock Breeding, 1900–2000 (Toronto: University of Toronto Press, 2020).

78 http://web.kwpn.nl, http://www.winsomestables.com/history.htm, accessed 17 November 2004.

79 For some general information on the Trakehner, the Hanoverian, and the Dutch Warmblood, see http://www.nawpn.org, http://web.kwpn.nl, http://www.winsomestables.com/history.htm, http://www.dutchharnesshorses.nl/Main1.php?S=TheBreed&SC=2&F=1&C=1&FC=5&…, http://web.kwpn.nl/html/newsletter, http://white_arabian.tripod.com/dutchwarmblood.html, http://imh.org/imh/bw/trak/html, http://www.imh.org/imh/bw/hanov.html, http://www.imh.org/imh/bw/dwarm.html, all accessed 17 November 2004.

80 *AHW*, May 2003, 236–7.

81 http://www.renaihorseregistry.com/message.asp, accessed 17 November 2004.

82 Ibid.

83 Ibid.; *AHW*, February 2003, 348–51.

84 *AHW*, July 2003, 89–96; November 2003, 144, 147.

85 See https://www.dandb.com/businessdirectory/therenaihorseregistryinc-lagrange-ky-15235613.html, accessed 30 April 2019.

86 https://equineprpro.blogspot.com/2008/02/interview-with-arabian-horse-icon-gene.html, accessed 30 April 2019.

87 *AHW*, April 2003, 178–9; May 2003, 6, 16; July 2003, 76–7.

88 Ibid., January 2003, 204–5.

89 Ibid., January 2003, 6.

90 Ibid., February 2003, 16.

91 Ibid., July 2003, 16, 312.

92 http://nshregistry.org/StaticPageDisp.asp?ID=33, accessed 30 April 2019.

8. The Effects of Pedigrees on International Trade

1 See M. Derry, *Ontario's Cattle Kingdom: Purebred Breeders and Their World, 1870–1920* (Toronto: University of Toronto Press, 2001), 71–83. See, for example, Sessional Paper 28, Legislature of Ontario (henceforth SP, Ontario), 1896, 175; *Canadian Live-Stock and Farm Journal*, February 1885, 31; January 1887, 65.

2 The situation in Canada with reference to government activity in purebred affairs differed from that in the United States. In effect, government after 1895 agreed to breeder control of standards and set up

a system by which those standards could be certified. The issue was more about pedigree accuracy than control for import reasons. For more on the Canadian situation, see M. Derry, *Bred for Perfection: Shorthorn Cattle, Collies, and Arabian Horses since 1800* (Baltimore: Johns Hopkins University Press, 2003), 33–44.

3 *Yearbook of the Department of Agriculture* (United States), 1913, 514.

4 A. Sanders, *Short-Horn Cattle: A Series of Historical Sketches, Memoirs and Records of the Breed and Its Development in the United States and Canada* (Chicago: Sanders, 1900), 282–3.

5 Sessional Paper 10, Parliament of Canada (henceforth SP, Canada), 1880, 119, 135, 138; SP 28, Ontario, 1896, Appendix D, "History of the Agriculture and Arts Association," 164, 174–5.

6 Ontario Agricultural Commission, 1881, vol. 3, Appendix G, 6.

7 Ibid., 19.

8 For more on this story, see M.E. Derry, *Ontario's Cattle Kingdom: Purebred Breeders and Their World, 1870–1920* (Toronto: University of Toronto Press, 2001), 53–85.

9 *Farmer's Advocate*, July 1881, 157; October 1881, 248; December 1881, 294; April 1886, 105–6. *Canadian Live-Stock and Farm Journal*, February 1886, 31; April 1887, 459.

10 See SP 10, Ontario, 1888, 55. An assessment of essays on prize farms, which were published in the Ontario Legislature's Sessional Papers in the late 1880s and 1890s, shows how wide the effects of the pedigree changes were.

11 US Department of Agriculture, *Reports*, 1906, 29; 156; 1908, 266–7; *Field and Fancy*, 4 August, 1906, 4.

12 Arthur Johnson to Fisher, 19 January 1901, Letterbook 5, Arthur Johnson Papers, Public Archives of Ontario; US Department of Agriculture, *Report*, 1908, 267.

13 SP 24, Ontario, 1905, 19.

14 It is important to note, however, that tariffs against incoming stock – cattle in particular – were instigated and removed by the United States over the years after 1913. What was so significant here was the particular emphasis on the status of purebred stock as set by the Dingley tariff. Regulating entry on the basis of purebred qualification was no longer part of the story after 1913. Duty-free status would not be dictated by pedigree acceptance.

15 Ontario Agricultural Commission, *Report*, 1881, vol. 1, 550–2.

16 Ontario Agricultural Commission, *Report*, 1881, vol. 1, 551; vol. 3, Appendix G, 47; SP 28, Ontario, 1896, Appendix D, 150.

17 *Farming*, September 1896, 21; SP 8, Ontario, 1889, 4–5.

18 SP 28, Ontario, 1899, 133, 141–7; SP 73, Ontario, 1899, 32–4.

19 *Breeder's Gazette*, 1 January 1890, 11.
20 The author thanks the University of Toronto Press for permission to reuse material that appears in a different and more comprehensive form in books written by her and published by the press.
21 K. Chivers, *The Shire Horse: A History of the Breed, the Society and the Men* (London: Routledge and Kegan Paul, 1976), 64–5.
22 *Breeder's Gazette*, 23 February 1882, 292. For more on the Clyde/Shire story and importing/exporting, see my *Horses in Society: A Story of Animal Breeding and Marketing Culture, 1800–1920* (Toronto: University of Toronto Press, 2006), 48–69.
23 *Breeder's Gazette*, 23 November 1882, 662.
24 *Stud Book of the Select Clydesdale Horse Society of Scotland*, vol. 1 (1883), xxxii.
25 E. Baird, *The Clydesdale Horse* (London: P.T. Batsford, 1982), 20–1, 26, 27–30; *Breeder's Gazette*, 10 August 1882, 213.
26 *Stud Book of the Select Clydesdale Horse Society of Scotland*, vol. 1 (1883), xvi.
27 Ibid., xx, xxi.
28 SP 12, Ontario, 1892, 5.
29 R.F. Moore-Colyer, "Aspects of Horse Breeding and the Supply of Horses in Victorian Britain," *Agriculture History Review* 43 (1995): 52.
30 *Canadian Live-Stock and Farm Journal*, February 1895, 55.
31 Ontario Agricultural Commission, vol. 3, Appendix H, 65.
32 "Minutes of Evidence taken before the Departmental Committee appointed to enquire and Report as the British Trade in Live Stock with the Colonies and Other Countries," 1912, Cd. 6032, 153, 154; Moore-Colyer, "Aspects of Horse Breeding," 54.
33 Ibid., 43–6; "Minutes of Evidence," Cd. 6032, 138, 153; G. MacEwan, *Heavy Horses: Highlights of Their History* (Saskatoon: Western Producer Prairie Books, 1986), 15. In spite of the falling-off of the market at the end of the 1880s, Canadian farmers continued to find it comparatively easy to sell their heavy drafters for use in US cities. See *Farmer's Advocate*, December 1889, 380.
34 MacEwan, *Heavy Horses*, 17; *Farmer's Advocate*, February 1890, 39; "The Canadian Draught Horse Stud Book," vol. 1 (Hunter, Rose & Co., Toronto, 1889), np.
35 MacEwan, *Heavy Horses*, 17; *Farmer's Advocate*, February 1890, 39; "The Canadian Draught Horse Stud Book," vol. 1, np. A second draft horse stud book for Shire/Clyde crosses was initiated in Goderich, Ontario. See *Canadian Live-Stock and Farm Journal*, July 1888, 100–1. The association that generated the pedigrees was forced out of business in 1906 after issuing four stud books. See *Farming World and Canadian Farm and Home*, 1 March 1906, 269.

36 *Breeder's Gazette*, 27 June 1888, 642.
37 *Farmer's Advocate*, October 1889, 308.
38 Ibid., July 1891, 247.
39 Ibid., December 1890, 396.
40 MacEwan, *Heavy Horses*, 42–3, 50–2; *Farmer's Advocate*, 7 November 1918, 1788; *Breeder's Gazette*, 5 March 1885, 357.
41 *Breeder's Gazette*, 8 November 1883, 640.
42 Ibid., 25 June 1885, 971.
43 Ibid., 12 February 1885, 239; 19 November 1885, 813; 10 March 1887, 381; 8 December 1887, 909–10; 28 March 1888, 317; 21 August 1889, 180; 12 February 1885, 239; 28 March 1888, 317.
44 Ibid., 4 January 1888, 13–14.
45 Ibid., 13 June 1888, 572.
46 Ibid., 17 November 1887, 795.
47 K. Voth, "From Big to Small to Big to Small: Part 2 of a Pictorial History of Cattle Changes over the Years," *On Pasture*, 11 July 2016, 1–2; based on the research of Harlan Ritchie of Michigan State University on the history of beef cattle styles. http://onpasture.com/2016/07/11/from-big-to-small-to-big-to-small-part-2-of-a-pictorial-history-of-cattle-changes-over-the-years, accessed 13 July 2016. See http://hansard.millbanksystems.com/commons/1963/apr/10/charolais-cattle-import
   HANSARD 1803–2005 → 1960s → 1963 → April 1963 → 10 April 1963 → Commons Sitting → WAYS AND MEANS [9th April] CHAROLAIS CATTLE (IMPORT) House of Commons Debates, 10 April 1963 vol. 675 cc 1437–48, 1437; and http://simmental-sbl.blogspot.ca/2011/12/about-this-blog.html; http://simmental-sbl.blogspot.ca/, accessed 30 October 2015; Don Vaniman, executive secretary of the American Simmental Association, *Simmental Shield*, August 1974, 119–22.
48 M. Derry, "Genetics, Biotechnology, and Breeding: North American Shorthorn Production in the 21st Century," *Agricultural History* 92 (Winter 2018).
49 http://www.steerplanet.com/bb/the-big-show/deerpark-leader-16th-and-d-seamus-4th/, accessed 10 May 2015.
50 http://www.steerplanet.com/bb/the-big-show/asterisk-free-shorthorn/?nowap, accessed 10 May 2015.
51 http://www.steerplanet.com/bb/the-big-show/deerpark-leader-16th-and-d-seamus-4th/, accessed 12 May 2015.
52 http://www.steerplanet.com/bb/the-big-show/asterisk-free-shorthorn/?nowap, accessed 13 June 2015.
53 http://www.steerplanet.com/bb/the-big-show/shorty-folks/45/, accessed 13 June 2015.

54 http://www.steerplanet.com/bb/the-big-show/deerpark-leader-13th/?nowap, accessed 10 May 2015.
55 http://www.steerplanet.com/bb/the-big-show/asterisk-free-shorthorn/?nowap, accessed 12 May 2015.
56 "With the International," *Arabian Horse News*, May 1959, 12; R. Archer et al., *The Crabbet Arabian Stud: Its History and Influence* (Northleach, UK: Alexander Heriot, 1978), 170. For more on Arabians, see Lady Wentworth (Judith Anne Blunt), *The Authentic Arabian Horse* (London: George Allen & Unwin, 1945); J. Forbis, *The Classic Arabian Horse* (New York: Liveright, 1976); C. Raswan, *The Arab and His Horse* (Oakland, CA: Raswan, 1955); H.H. Reese, *The Kellogg Arabians: Their Background and Influence* (Alhambra, CA: Bordon, 1958); Lady Anne Blunt, *A Pilgrimage to Nejd* (1881; reprint London: Century Publishing Co., 1985); W.S. Blunt, *My Diaries*, vol. 1 [1888–1900] and vol. 2 [1900–14] (London: Ernest Benn, 1927); D. Landry, *Noble Brutes: How Eastern Culture Transformed English Culture* (Baltimore: Johns Hopkins University Press, 2009).
57 "Breeders of the Northeast: A Look Back," *Arabian Horse World* (henceforth *AHW*), November 1988, 143–4; "Davenport Arabian Horses," *Arabiana*, 1–5; M. Bowling, "The CMK Heritage," http://www.dsrtweyr.com/cmk/cmkmbheritage.html, accessed 28 August 1999.
58 "Registration Certificates," *Arab Horse Journal* (henceforth *AHJ*), March 1960, 8.
59 "Mission & History," *The Registry*, http://www.theregistry.org/mission/index.shtml.
60 *AHW*, June 1987, 410. See also *AHJ*, March 1961, 31, 37.
61 WAHO Publication no. 21, Part 4, "AHRA Importation Policies & History," http://www.euroarab.com/news/excerpt4.htm, accessed 24 August 1999. This document is supported by evidence from many archival sources.
62 WAHO Publication 21, Part 5, "Purity Wasn't the Issue at All," http://www.waho.org/Purityissue.html, accessed 28 August 1999.
63 WAHO Publication 21, Part 4, "AHRA Importation Policies & History," http://www.waho.org/Purityissue.html 28 August 1999, accessed 12 December 2001.
64 *AHW*, September 1980, 241, 243; August 1985, 289–90.
65 Ibid., July 1986, 404–5.
66 Ibid., April 1986, 237, 240, 241.
67 Ibid., March 1987, 191, 194.
68 *The Arabian* 1 (1974): 18.
69 *AHW*, July 1986, 406.
70 Ibid., August 1985, 290.

71 WAHO publication 21, "Is Purity the Issue?" http://www.waho.org/Purity.html, accessed 26 September 1999. This long document contains many sections that were useful.
72 *The Arabian* 1 (1974): 18.
73 Letter, http://euroarab.com/news/aha/htm, accessed 24 August 1999.
74 "AHRA and Jordan Sign … Agreement," press release, *The Registry*, 13 February 1998, http://www.theregistry.org/press/pr980213.shtml, accessed 24 August 1999.
75 "Questions and Answers – Alliance of the Americas," press release, *The Registry*, 6 October 2001, http://www.theregistry.org/News/PressReleasesView.asp?id=11, accessed 12 December 2001.
76 See C. Lange, "Purity, Nobility, Beauty and Performance: Past and Present Construction of Meaning for the Arabian Horse," in *The Meaning of Horses: Biosocial Encounters*, ed. D.L. Davis and A. Maustad (London: Routledge Press, 2016), 39–53, and his "The Making and Remaking of the Arabian Horse – from the Arab Bedouin Horse to the Modern Straight Egyptian," in *Horse Breeds and Human Society: Purity, Identity and the Making of the Modern Horse*, ed. K. Guest and M. Mattfeld (London: Routledge Press, 2020), 234–51.
77 J. Forbis, *Authentic Arabian Boodstock II: The Story of Ansata and Sharing the Dream* (Mena, AR: Ansata Publishing, 2003), 28.
78 See Lange, "Purity, Nobility, Beauty and Performance," esp. 48–50.
79 See Derry, *Bred for Perfection*, 17–47.

Final Remarks

1 Interview with Dominic Elfick, geneticist for the poultry breeder company Aviagen, 24–5 May 2007.

Selected Bibliography of Useful Sources

Books

Abott, H. "The Marketing of Livestock in Canada." MA thesis, University of Toronto, 1923.

Anderson, V.D. *Creatures of Empire: How Domestic Animals Transformed Early America*. Oxford: Oxford University Press, 2004.

Arabiana: An Anthology of Articles about Arabian Horses and Their Owners Reprinted from "Your Pony" and "The International Rider and Driver" – 1959 to 1974. Fort Atkinson, WI: Bill Simpson, 1975.

Archer, R., C. Pearson, and C. Govey. *The Crabbet Arabian Stud: Its History and Influence*. Northleach, UK: Alexander Heriot, 1978.

Atack, J., and F. Bateman. *To Their Own Soil: Agriculture in the Antebellum North*. Ames: Iowa State University Press, 1987.

Bajema, C.J., ed. *Artificial Selection and the Development of Evolutionary Theory*. Stroudsburg, PA: Hutchinson Ross Publishing, 1982.

Barclay, H.H. *The Role of the Horse in Human Culture*. London: J.A. Allen, 1980.

Barnes, D., ed. *The AKC's World of the Pure-Bred Dog*. Cambridge, MA: Basil Blackwell, 1990.

Bates, C.J. *Thomas Bates and the Kirklevington Shorthorns: A Contribution to the History of Pure Durham Cattle*. Newcastle upon Tyne: Robert Redpath, 1897.

Beauchamp, T.L., et al. *The Human Use of Animals: Case Studies in Ethical Practice*. Oxford: Oxford University Press, 2008.

Bennett, O.P., and T.M. Halpin. *The Collie*. Washington, IL: O.P. Bennett, 1942.

Bidwell, P.W., and J.L. Falconer. *History of Agriculture in the Northern United States*. Washington, DC: Carnegie Institute, 1925.

Blunt, Lady Anne. *A Pilgrimage to Nejd*. 1881. Reprint London: Century Publishing Company, 1985.

Bogue, A. *From Prairie to Corn Belt: Farming on the Illinois and Iowa Prairies in the Nineteenth Century*. Chicago: University of Chicago Press, 1963.

Bourdon, R.M. *Understanding Animal Breeding*. 2nd edition. Upper Saddle River, NJ: Prentice Hall, 2000.

Bowler, P.J. *The Eclipse of Darwinism, Anti-Darwinism Evolutionary Theories in the Decades around 1900*. Baltimore: Johns Hopkins University Press, 1983,

– *The History of an Idea*. Berkeley: University of California Press, 1984

– *The Non-Darwinian Revolution: Reinterpreting a Historical Myth*. Baltimore: Johns Hopkins University Press, 1988.

Brackett, B.G., et al, eds. *New Technologies in Animal Breeding*. New York: Academic Press, 1981.

Brown, W.R. *The Horse of the Desert*. New York: Macmillan Company, 1929, reprint 1947.

Bulmer, M. *Francis Galton: Pioneer of Heredity and Biometry*. Baltimore: Johns Hopkins University Press, 2003.

Caras, R.A. *Going for the Blue: Inside the World of Show Dogs and Dog Shows*. New York: Warner Books, 2001.

Cassidy, R. *Horse People: Thoroughbred Culture in Lexington and Newmarket*. Baltimore: Johns Hopkins University Press, 2007.

– *The Sport of Kings: Kinship, Class and Thoroughbred Breeding in Newmarket*. Cambridge: Cambridge University Press, 2002.

Castle, W.E. *Heredity in Relation to Evolution and Animal Breeding*. New York: D. Appleton and Company, 1911.

Chapman, A.B., ed. *General and Quantitative Genetics*. Amsterdam: Elsevier Science Publishers, 1985.

Chivers, K. *The Shire Horse, A History of the Breed, the Society and the Men*. London: Routledge and Kegan Paul, 1976.

Clausen, R.E. *Genetics in Relation to Agriculture*. New York: McGraw-Hill Book Company, 1918.

Coleman, W., and C. Limoges, eds. *Studies in History of Biology*. Baltimore: Johns Hopkins University Press, 1979.

Collie Club of America. *The Complete Collie*. New York: Howell Book House, 1962.

Comstock, R.E. *Quantitative Genetics with Special Reference to Plant and Animal Breeding*. Ames: Iowa State University Press, 1996.

Cox, L. "'Reasonable Tact and Diplomacy': Disease Management and Bovine Tuberculosis in North America, 1890–1950." PhD thesis, University of Guelph, 2013.

Crawford, R.D., ed. *Poultry Breeding and Genetics*. New York: Elsevier, 1990.

Crow, J.F. *Basic Concepts in Population, Quantitative, and Evolutionary Genetics*. New York: W.H. Freeman and Company, 1986.

Culley, G. *Observations on Live Stock: containing hints for choosing and improving the best breeds of the most useful kinds of domestic animals*. London: D. Longworth, 1804.

Cunningham, E.P. *Quantitative Genetic Theory and Livestock Improvement.* Armidale, NSW: University of New England, 1979.
Dalziel, H. *British Dogs: Describing the History, Characteristics, Points, and Club Standards, of the Various Breeds of Dogs Established in Great Britain,* volume 2. 2nd edition. London: L. Upcott Gill, 1889.
– *The Collie: Its History, Points, and Breeding.* London: L. Upcott Gill, 1888.
Derry, M.E. *Art and Science in Breeding: Creating Better Chickens.* Toronto: University of Toronto Press, 2012.
– *Bred for Perfection: Shorthorn Cattle, Collies, and Arabian Horses since 1800.* Baltimore: Johns Hopkins University Press, 2003.
– *Horses in Society: A Story of Breeding and Marketing Culture, 1800–1920.* Toronto: University of Toronto Press, 2006.
– *Masterminding Nature: The Breeding of Animals, 1750–2010.* Toronto: University of Toronto Press, 2015.
– *Ontario's Cattle Kingdom: Purebred Breeders and Their World, 1870–1920.* Toronto: University of Toronto Press, 2001.
Dreyer, P. *A Gardener Touched with Genius.* Los Angeles: University of California Press, 1985.
Dunn, L.C. *A Short History of Genetics: The Development of Some of the Main Lines of Thought, 1864–1939.* New York: McGraw-Hill, 1965.
Dunn, L.C., ed. *Genetics in the 20th Century.* New York: Macmillan Company, 1951.
Ensminger, E.M. *Beef Cattle Science.* Danville: Interstate Printers and Publishers, 1987.
Falconer, D.S. *Introduction to Quantitative Genetics.* Edinburgh: Oliver and Boyd, 1960.
Falk, R. *Genetic Analysis: A History of Genetic Thinking.* Cambridge: Cambridge University Press, 2009.
Felch, I.K. *The Breeding and Management of Poultry.* Hyde Park, NY: Norfolk County Press, 1877.
– *Poultry Culture: How to Raise, Mate and Judge Thoroughbred Fowls.* Chicago: Donohue, Henneberry, 1902.
Fitzgerald, D. *The Business of Breeding: Hybrid Corn in Illinois, 1890–1940.* Ithaca: Cornell University Press, 1990.
– *Every Farm a Factory.* New Haven: Yale University Press, 2003.
Forbis, J. *The Classic Arabian Horse.* New York: Liveright, 1976.
Fraser, A. *Animal Husbandry Heresies.* London: Crosby Lockwood & Son, 1960.
Freeman, S., and J.C. Herron. *Evolutionary Analysis.* Upper Saddle River, NJ: Prentice Hall, 1998.
Frolov, I.T. *Philosophy and History of Genetics: The Inquiry and the Debates.* London: Macdonald, 1991.

Fudge, E. *Perceiving Animals: Humans and Beasts in Early Modern English Culture*. Basingstoke: Macmillan Press, 2000.
Futuyma, D.F. *Evolutionary Biology*. 3rd edition. Sunderland, MA. Sinauer Associates, 1998.
Gaudillière, Jean-Paul, et al., eds. *From Molecular Genetics to Genomics: The Mapping Cultures of the Twentieth Century*. London: Routledge, 2004.
Gianola, D., et al., eds. *Advances in Statistical Methods for Genetic Improvement of Livestock*. Berlin: Springer-Verlag, 1990.
Gillham, N.R. *A Life of Sir Francis Galton: From African Exploration to the Birth of Eugenics*. Oxford: Oxford University Press, 2001.
Glass, B., O. Temkin, and W.L. Straus Jr., eds. *Forerunners of Darwin, 1745–1859*. Baltimore: Johns Hopkins University Press, 1951.
Goodall, D.M. *A History of Horse Breeding*. London: Robert Hall, 1977.
Greely, M. *Arabian Exodus*. London: J.A. Allen, 1975.
Green, E.L. *Genetics and Probability in Animal Breeding Experiments*. London: Macmillan, 1981.
Grothe, P.O. *Holstein Friesian: A Global Breed*. Netherlands: Misset Press, 1993 (English version 1994).
Guest, K., and M. Mattfeld, eds. *Horse Breeds and Human Society: Purity, Identity and the Making of the Modern Horse*. London: Routledge Press, 2020.
Hagedoorn, A.L. *Animal Breeding*. London: Crosby Lockwood & Son, 1939; 6th edition 1962.
Hagedoorn, A.L., and G. Skyes. *Poultry Breeding: Theory and Practice*. London: Crosby Lockwood & Son, 1953.
Hanke, O.A., ed. *American Poultry History, 1823–1973*. Madison, WI: American Poultry History Society, 1974.
Harman, O., and M.R. Dietrich, eds. *Rebels, Mavericks, and Heretics in Biology*. New Haven: Yale University Press, 2008.
Harper, M.H. *Breeding of Farm Animals*. New York: Orange Judd Company, 1920.
Hartl, D.L. *A Primer of Population Genetics*. Sunderland, MA: Sinauer Associates, 1981.
Harwood, J. *Styles of Scientific Thought: The German Genetics Community, 1900–1933*. Chicago: University of Chicago Press, 1992.
– *Technology's Dilemma: Agricultural Colleges between Science and Practice in Germany, 1860–1934*. New York: Peter Lang Publishing Group, 2005.
Hayes, F.A., and G.T. Klein. *Poultry Breeding Applied*. Mount Morris, IL: Watt Publishing Company, 1952.
Hemsworth, P.H., and G.J. Coleman. *Human-Livestock Interactions: The Stockperson and the Productivity and Welfare of Intensively Farmed Animals*. London: CAB International, 1998.

Herman, H.A. *Improving Cattle by the Millions: NAAB and the Development and Worldwide Application of Artificial Insemination*. Columbia: University of Missouri Press, 1981.

Hill, W.G., and T.F.C. Mackay, eds. *Evolution and Animal Breeding: Reviews on Molecular and Quantitative Approaches in Honour of Alan Robertson*, Wallingford, UK: C.A.B. International, 1989.

Housman, W. *The Improved Shorthorn: Notes and Reflections upon Some Facts in Shorthorn History, with Remarks upon Certain Principles of Breeding*. London: Ridgeway, 1876.

Hutt, F.D., and B.A. Rasmusen. *Animal Genetics*. 2nd edition. New York: John Wiley & Sons, [1964] 1982.

Innis, H., ed. *The Dairy Industry in Canada*. Toronto: Ryerson Press, 1937.

Introduction to Molecular Genetics and Genomics. www.bio-nica.info/biblioteca/AnonimoxxxIntroductionMolecularGEnetics.pdf.

Jaquet, E.W. *The Kennel Club: A History and Record of Its Work*. London: Kennel Gazette, 1905.

Johnson, P.C. *Farm Animals in the Making of America*. Des Moines: Wallace Homestead Book Company, 1975.

Jones, R. *History of Agriculture in Ohio to 1880*. Kent, OH: Kent State University Press, 1983.

Jordan, T. *North American Cattle Ranching Frontiers: Origins, Diffusion, and Differentiation*. Histories of the American Frontier. Albuquerque: University of New Mexico Press, 1993.

Jull, A. *Poultry Breeding*. 3rd edition. New York: John Wiley & Sons, 1952.

Kaye, G. *The Collie in America*. Valley Center, CA: Chelsea, 2008.

Kingsland, S.E. *Modeling Nature: Episodes in the History of Population Ecology*. Chicago: University of Chicago Press, 1995.

Kitcher, P. *In Mendel's Mirror*. Oxford: Oxford University Press, 2003.

Kloppenburg, J.R. *First the Seed: The Political Economy of Plant Biotechnology, 1492–2000*. Cambridge: Cambridge University Press, 1988.

Kuhn, T.S. *The Essential Tension*. Chicago: University of Chicago Press, 1977.

– *The Structure of Scientific Revolutions*. 4th edition. Chicago: University of Chicago Press, 2012.

Lampard, E.E. *The Rise of the Dairy Industry in Wisconsin: A Study of Agricultural Change, 1820–1920*. Madison: State Historical Society of Wisconsin, 1963.

Lerner, I.M. *The Genetic Basis of Selection*. New York: John Wiley & Sons, 1958.

– *Population Genetics and Animal Improvement*. Cambridge: Cambridge University Press, 1950.

Lerner, I.M., and H. Donald. *Modern Developments in Animal Breeding*. London and New York: Academic Press, 1966.

Lush, J. *Animal Breeding Plans*. Ames, IA: Collegiate Press, 1937.

MacEwan, G. *Highlights of Shorthorn History*. Winnipeg: Hignill Printing, 1982.

Mansfield, R.H. *Progress of the Breed: The History of U.S. Holsteins*. Holstein-Friesian World, 1985.

Marcus, A.I. *Agricultural Science and the Quest for Legitimacy: Farmers, Agricultural Colleges, and Experiment Stations, 1870–1890*. Ames: Iowa State University Press, 1985.

Marcus Porcius Cato on Agriculture; Marcus Terentius Varro on Agriculture. Revised by H.B. Ash, translated by W.D. Hooper. Cambridge, MA: Harvard University Press, 1934, reprint 1960.

Marie, J. "The Importance of Place: A History of Genetics in 1930s Britain." PhD thesis, University College London, 2004.

Marshall, K. *His Dogs: Albert Payson Terhune and the Sunnybank Collies*. New York: Collie Club of America [Collie Health Foundation], 2001.

Matz, B. "Crafting Heredity: The Art and Science of Livestock Breeding in the United States and Germany, 1860–1914." PhD thesis, Yale University, December 2011.

Mayr, E., and W.B. Provine. *The Evolutionary Synthesis: Perspectives on the Unification of Biology*. Cambridge, MA: Harvard University Press, 1980.

Mazumdar, P.M.H. *Eugenics, Human Genetics and Human Failings: The Eugenics Society, Its Sources and Critics in Britain*. London: Routledge, 1992.

– *Species and Specificity: An Interpretation of the History of Immunology*. Cambridge: Cambridge University Press, 1995.

McCormick, V. *Farm Wife: A Self-Portrait, 1886–1896*. Ames: Iowa State University, 1990.

McElheny, V.K. *Watson and DNA: Making a Scientific Revolution*. New York: Perseus Publishing, 2003.

McMurry, S. *Transforming Rural America: Dairying Families and Agricultural Change, 1820–1885*. Baltimore: Johns Hopkins University Press, 1995.

Mingay, G., ed. *Arthur Young and His Times*. London: Macmillan Press, 1975.

Montcrieff, E., S. Joseph, and I. Joseph. *Farm Animal Portraits*, Woodbridge, UK: Antique Collectors' Club, 1996.

Morwick, E.Y. *The Chosen Breed: A Tale of Men, Women and the Canadian Holstein*. 2 vols. Hamilton, ON: Printed by Seldon Griffin Graphics, 2002.

Müller-Wille, S., and H.J. Rheinberger. *A Cultural History of Heredity*. Chicago: University of Chicago Press, 2012, reprint 2014.

Olby, R. *Origins of Mendelism*. 2nd edition. Chicago: University of Chicago Press, 1985.

Olson, A., and J. Voss. *The Organization of Knowledge in America, 1860–1920*. Baltimore: Johns Hopkins University Press, 1979.

Orde, A., ed. *Mathew and George Culley: Travel Journals and Letters, 1765–1798*. Oxford: Oxford University Press, 2002.

Packwood, H.E. *Show Collies: Rough and Smooth Coated, A Complete History*. Np, 1906.

Pawson, H.C. *Robert Bakewell: Pioneer Livestock Breeder*. London: Crosby Lockwood, 1957.

Persell, S.M. *Neo-Lamarckism and the Evolution Controversy in France, 1870–1920*. Lewiston: Edwin Mellen Press, 1999.

Pirchner, F. *Population Genetics in Animal Breeding*. San Francisco: W.H. Freeman and Company, 1969.

Pollak, E., et al., eds. *Proceedings of the International Conference on Quantitative Genetics*. Ames: Iowa State University Press, 1977.

Powell, F.W. *Bureau of Animal Industry: Its History, and Organization*. New York: AMS Press, 1974.

Provine, W.B. *The Origins of Theoretical Population Genetics*. Chicago: University of Chicago Press, 1971.

– *Sewall Wright and Evolutionary Biology*. Chicago: University of Chicago Press, 1986.

Quirk, L. *Prof William Richard Graham: Poultryman of the Century*. Guelph: University of Guelph, 2005.

Rader, K. *Making Mice: Standardizing Animals for American Biomedical Research, 1900–1955*. Princeton: Princeton University Press, 2004.

Reaman, G.E. *History of the Holstein-Friesian Breed in Canada*. Toronto: Collins, 1946.

Reese, H.H. *The Kellogg Arabians: Their Background and Influence*. Alhambra, CA: Bordon Publishing Company, 1958.

Rheinberger, H.J., and S. Müller-Wille. *The Gene: From Genetics to Postgenomics*. Translated by A. Bostanci. Chicago: University of Chicago Press, 2017.

Richardson S., and H. Stevens, eds. *Postgenomics*. Durham, NC: Duke University Press, 2015.

Rifkin, J. *Beyond Beef: The Rise and Fall of the Cattle Culture*. New York: Penguin Books, 1992.

Ritvo, H. *The Animal Estate*. Cambridge, MA: Harvard University Press, 1987.

– *The English and Other Creatures in the Victorian Age*. Cambridge, MA: Harvard University Press, 1987.

– *The Platypus and the Mermaid and Other Figments of the Classifying Imagination*. Cambridge, MA: Harvard University Press, 1997.

Rogers, E.M. *Diffusion of Innovations*. New York: Free Press of Glencoe, 1962.

Rossiter, M. *The Emergence of Agricultural Science*. New Haven: Yale University Press, 1975.

Rothschild, M., and S. Newman, eds. *Intellectual Property Rights in Animal Breeding and Genetics*. New York: CABI Publishing, 2002.

Russell, E. *Greyhound Nation: A Coevolutionary History of England, 1200–1900*. Cambridge: Cambridge University Press, 2018.

Russell, N. *Like Engend'ring Like: Heredity and Animal Breeding in Early Modern England*. Cambridge: Cambridge University Press, 1986.
Ryder, M.L. *Sheep and Man*. London: Duckworth, 1983.
Sanders, A. *Red, White and Roan*. Chicago: American Shorthorn Breeders' Association, 1936.
– *Short-Horn Cattle, a Series of Historical Sketches, Memoirs and Records of the Breed and Its Development in the United States and Canada*. Chicago: Sanders Publishing, 1900.
Sanders, J.H. *The Breeds of Live Stock, and the Principles of Heredity*. Chicago: J.H. Sanders Publishing Company, 1887.
Sapp, J. *Beyond the Gene: Cytoplasmic Inheritance and the Struggle for Authority in Genetics*. Oxford: Oxford University Press, 1987.
Sawyer, G. *The Agribusiness Poultry Industry: A History of Its Development*. New York: Exposition Press, 1971.
Schapsmeier, E.L., and F.H. Schapsmeier. *Henry A. Wallace of Iowa: The Agrarian Years, 1910–1940*. Ames: Iowa State University Press, 1968.
Scott, R. *The Reluctant Farmer: The Rise of Agricultural Extension to 1914*. Chicago: University of Chicago Press, 1970.
Serafini, A. *The Epic History of Biology*. New York: Plenum Press, 1993.
Serpell, J., ed. *In the Company of Animals: A Study of Human-Animal Relations*. Cambridge: Cambridge University Press, 1996.
Shaw, T. *Animal Breeding*. Chicago: Orange Judd Company, 1901.
– *The Study of Breeds*. Chicago: Orange Judd Company, 1900.
Shepard, P. *The Others: How Animals Made Us Human*. Washington, DC: Island Press, 1995.
Shreeve, J. *The Genome War: How Craig Venter Tried to Capture the Code of Life and Save the World*. New York: Alfred A. Knopf, 2004.
Simm, G. *Genetic Improvement of Cattle and Sheep*. Ipswich: Farming Press, 1998.
Smocovitis, V.B. *Unifying Biology: The Evolutionary Synthesis and Evolutionary Biology*. Princeton: Princeton University Press, 1996.
Snyder, E.S. "A History of the Poultry Science Department at the Ontario Agricultural College, 1894–1968." Unpublished manuscript, 1970.
Sturtevant, A.H. *A History of Genetics*. New York: Cold Spring Harbor Laboratory Press, 1964, reprint 2001.
Swart, S., and G. Bankoff, eds. *Breeds of Empire: The "Invention" of the Horse in Southeast Asia and Southern Africa*. Copenhagen: Nordic Institute of Asian Studies Press, 2007.
Tesio, F. *Tesio: In His Own Words*. Translated by M. Burnett. Neenah, WI: Russell Meerdink Company, 2005. Original version: *Puro-Sangue – Animale da Experimento*. Milan: Ulrico Hoepli, 1947.
Theunissen, L.T.G. *Beauty or Statistics: Practice and Science in Dutch Livestock Breeding, 1900–2000*. Toronto: University of Toronto Press, 2020.

Thomas, K. *Man and the Natural World: Changing Attitudes in England 1500–1800*. London: Allen Lane, 1983.
Thompson, J.A. *History of Livestock Raising in the United States, 1607–1860*. Washington, DC: Bureau of Agricultural Economics, 1942.
Thurtle, P. *The Emergence of Genetic Rationality: Space, Time and Transformation in American Biological Science, 1870–1920*. Seattle: University of Washington Press, 2008.
Trow-Smith, R. *A History of British Livestock Husbandry, 1700–1900*. London: Routledge and Kegan Paul, 1959.
Tudge, C. *In Mendel's Footnotes: An Introduction to the Science and Technologies of Genes and Genetics from the Nineteenth Century to the Twenty-Second*. London: Jonathan Cape, 2000.
Walsh, J. (Stonehenge). *The Greyhound in 1864: Breeding, Rearing, and Training of Greyhounds*. London: Longman, Green, Longman, Roberts & Green, 1864.
Ward, Peter. *Lamarck's Revenge: How Epigenetics Is Revolutionizing Our Understanding of Evolution's Past and Present*. New York: Bloomsbury Publishing, 2018.
Warren, D.C. *Practical Poultry Breeding*. New York: Macmillan Company, 1953.
Weir, B.S., et al., eds. *Proceedings of the Second International Conference on Quantitative Genetics*. Sunderland, MA: Sinauer Associates, 1988.
Wentworth, Lady (Judith Anne Blunt). *The Authentic Arabian Horse*. London: George Allen & Unwin, 1945.
– *Thoroughbred Racing Stock*. New York: Charles Scribner's Sons, 1938.
– *Toy Dogs and Their Ancestors*. London: Duckworth, 1911.
Wood, R.J., and V. Orel. *Genetic Prehistory in Selective Breeding: A Prelude to Mendel*. Oxford: Oxford University Press, 2001.
Woods, R. *The Herds Shot around the World: Native Breeds and the British Empire, 1800–1900*. Chapel Hill: University of North Carolina Press, 2017.
Worboys, M., J.-M. Strange, and N. Pemberton. *The Invention of the Modern Dog: Breed and Blood in Victorian Britain*. Baltimore: Johns Hopkins University Press, 2018.
Wriedt, C. *Heredity in Live Stock*. London: Macmillan and Company, 1930.

Articles

Allen, G.E. "Mendelian Genetics and Postgenomics: The Legacy for Today." *Ludus Vitalis* 21 (2004): 213–36.
Alter, S.G. "The Advantages of Obscurity: Charles Darwin's Negative Inference from the History of Domestic Breeds." *Annals of Science* 64 (2007): 235–50.
Andersson, L. "Genome-Wide Association Analysis in Domestic Animals: A Powerful Approach for Genetic Dissection of Trait Loci." *Genetica* 136 (2009): 341–9.

Ashwell, M.S., et al. "A Genome Scan to Identify Quantitative Trait Loci Affecting Economically Important Traits in a US Holstein Population." *Journal of Dairy Science* 84 (2001): 2535–42.

Barendse, W. "Development and Commercialization of a Genetic Marker for Marbling of Beef in Cattle: A Case Study." In *Intellectual Property Rights in Animal Breeding and Genetics*, edited by M. Rothschild and S. Newman, 197–212. New York: CABI Publishing, 2002.

Barker, J.S.F. "Quantitative Genetics, Ecology, and Evolution." *Proceedings of the Second International Conference on Quantitative Genetics*, edited by B.S. Weir, 596–600. Sunderland, MA: Sinauer Associates, 1988.

Bateman, F. "Improvement in American Dairy Farming, 1850–1910: A Quantitative Analysis." *Journal of Economic History* 28 (1968): 255–73.

– "Labor Inputs and Productivity in American Dairying, 1850–1910." *Journal of Economic History* 29 (1969): 206–29.

Beattie, C.W. "Development of Detailed Microsatellite Linkage Maps in Livestock." In *Biotechnology's Role in the Genetic Improvement of Farm Animals*, edited by R.H. Miller et al., 51–60. Beltsville Symposia in Agricultural Research, American Society of Animal Science, 1996.

Beckett, J.V. "Note on *Mathew and George Culley: Travel Journals and Letters, 1765–1798.*" *English Historical Review* 118 (2003): 803–4.

Bell, A.E. "Heritability in Retrospect." *Journal of Heredity* 68 (1977): 297–300.

Bichard, M. "Changes in Quantitative Genetic Technology in Animal Breeding." *Proceedings of the Second International Conference on Quantitative Genetics*, edited by B.S. Weir, 145–9. Sunderland, MA: Sinauer Associates, 1988.

Blackman, J. "The Cattle Trade and Agrarian Change on the Eve of the Railway Age." *Agriculture History Review* 23 (1975): 48–62.

Boniface, K. "Manufacturing the Horse: Understandings and Inheritance in the Long Eighteenth Century." In *Horse Breeds and Human Society: Purity, Identity and the Making of the Modern Horse*, edited by Kristen Guest and Monica Hattfeld, 50–66. London: Routledge Press, 2020.

Bonneuil, C. "Mendelism, Plant Breeding and Experimental Cultures: Agriculture and the Development of Genetics in France." *Journal of the History of Biology* 39 (2006): 281–308.

Bowie, G.G.S. "New Sheep for Old: Changes in Sheep Farming in Hampshire, 1792–1879." *Agricultural History Review* 35 (1987): 15–23.

Bowler, P.J. "The Changing Meaning of 'Evolution.'" *Journal of the History of Ideas* 36 (1975): 95–104.

Bowling, A.T., et al. "A Pedigree-Based Study of Mitochondrial d-Loop DNA Sequence Variation among Arabian Horses." *Animal Genetics* 31 (2000): 1–7.

Brassley, P. "Cutting across Nature? The History of Artificial Insemination of Pigs in the United Kingdom." *Studies in History and Philosophy of Biological and Biomedical Sciences* 38 (2007): 442–61.

Bresalier, M., and Michael Worboys. "'Saving the Lives of Our Dogs': The Development of Canine Distemper Vaccine in Interwar Britain." *British Journal for the History of Science* 47 (2014): 305–34.

Brunger, E. "Dairying and Urban Development in New York State, 1850–1900." *Agricultural History* 29 (1955): 169–73.

Bugos, G.E. "Intellectual Property Protection in the American Chicken-Breeding Industry." *Business History Review* 66 (1992): 127–68.

Bulmer, M. "Galton's Law of Ancestral Heredity." *Heredity* 81 (1998): 579–85.

Burke, J. "Dairywomen and Affectionate Wives: Women in the Irish Dairy Industry, 1890–1914." *Agricultural History Review* 38 (1990): 149–65.

Carlson, L. "Forging His Own Path: William Jasper Spillman and Progressive Era Breeding and Genetics." *Agricultural History* 79 (2005): 50–73.

Cassidy, R. "Falling in Love with Horses: The International Thoroughbred Auction." *Society and Animals* 13 (2005): 51–67.

– "Turf Wars: Arab Dimensions to British Racehorse Breeding." *Anthropology Today* 19 (2003): 13–18.

Castonguay, S. "The Transformation of Agricultural Research in France: The Introduction of the American System." *Minerva* 43 (2005): 265–87.

Chapman, A.B. "Jay Lawrence Lush 1896–1982: A Brief Biography." *Journal of American Science* 69 (1991): 2671–6.

Churchill, R.B. "William Johannsen and the Genotype Concept." *Journal of the History of Biology* 7 (1974): 5–30.

Clutton-Brock, J. "Darwin and the Domestication of Animals." *Biologist* 29 (1982): 72–6.

Cooke, K.J. "From Science to Practice, or Practice to Science? Chickens and Eggs in Raymond Pearl's Agricultural Breeding Research, 1907–1916." *Isis* 88 (1997): 62–86.

Copus, A.K. "Changing Markets and the Development of Sheep Breeds in Southern England, 1750–1900." *Agricultural History Review* 37 (1999): 238–51.

Cornell, J.F. "Analogy and Technology in Darwin's Vision of Nature." *Journal of the History of Biology* 17 (1984): 202–344.

Crew, F.A.E. "Reginald Crundall Punnett." *Genetics* 58 (1968): 1–7.

Crow, J.F. "Sewall Wright's Place in Twentieth-Century Biology." *Journal of the History of Biology* 23 (1990): 57–89.

Crow, J.R. Book review of *Proceedings of the Second International Conference on Quantitative Genetics* by B.S. Weir et al., 1988, in *Science* 242 (1988): 1449–50.

Davis, B.D. "The Background: Classical to Molecular Genetics." In *The Genetic Revolution: Scientific Prospects and Public Perceptions*, edited by B.D. Davis. Baltimore: Johns Hopkins University Press, 1991.

Denison, R.F., E.T. Kiers, and S.A. West. "Darwinian Agriculture: When Can Humans Find Solutions beyond the Reach of Natural Selection?" *Quarterly Journal of Biology* 78 (2003): 145–68.

Derry, M.E. "Chicken Breeding: The Complex Transition from Traditional to Genetic Methods in the United States." In *Cultivating Knowledge: New Perspectives on the History of Life Sciences and Agriculture*, edited by Sharon Kingsland and Denise Phillips. Archimedes series. New York: Springer, 2015.

– "Gender Conflicts in Dairying: Ontario's Butter Industry, 1880–1920." *Ontario History* 90 (1998): 31–47.

– "Genetics, Biotechnology, and Breeding: North American Shorthorn Production in the 21st Century." *Agricultural History* 92 (Winter 2018): 54–77.

– "Patterns of Gendered Labour and the Development of Ontario Agriculture." In *Ontario since Confederation: A Reader*, edited by E. Montigny and L. Chambers. Toronto: University of Toronto Press, 2000.

– "The Role of Purebred Breeder/Ordinary Farmer Conflict in the Rate of Herd Improvement – A Study of Cattle Farming in Ontario, 1870–1920." *Proceedings* for the Association of Living Historical Farms and Agricultural Museums Conference, 1998.

– "Theory and Method: An Analysis of European and American Animal Breeding Practices, 18th to 21st Century." *Agricultural History* 92 (2020): 324–61.

– "The Transition from Type to Breed: Draft Horses and Purebred Breeding in the International American Market, 1870–1920." In *Horse Breeds and Human Society: Purity, Identity and the Making of the Modern Horse*, edited by Kristen Guest and Monica Hattfeld, 195–212. London: Routledge Press, 2020.

– "White Collies, Beauty or Genetic Defect: Regulation and Breeding, 1870–2013." *Society and Animals* 28 (2020): 472–88.

Derry, M.E., B. Lightman, and R. Ankey. "The Commercialization of Breeding for Beauty." In book forum review on *The Invention of the Modern Dog: Breed and Blood in Victorian Britain*, by M. Worboys, Julie-Marie Strange, and Neil Pemberton. *Studies in History and Philosophy of Science* 84 (2020).

Driessen, C. "Deliberating with Crispr Creatures – When Bioethics Becomes a Matter of More-Than-Human/Cultural Geography." Unpublished paper, Uppsala University, Sweden, May 2018.

Dunn, L.C. "Genetics at the Anikowo Station: A Russian Animal Breeding Center That Has Been Developed during the Reconstruction Period." *Journal of Heredity* 19 (1928): 281–4.

– "The Transformation of Biology: A Geneticist's Viewpoint." *Journal of Heredity* 57 (1966): 159–65.

Evans, L.T. "Darwin's Use of the Analogy between Artificial and Natural Selection." *Journal of the History of Biology* 17 (1984): 113–40.

Falconer, D.S. "Early Selection Experiments." *Annual Review of Genetics* 26 (1992): 1–14.

– "Quantitative Genetics in Edinburgh, 1947–1980." *Genetics* 133 (1993): 137–42.

Froggatt, P., and N.C. Nevin. "Galton's 'Law of Ancesrtal Heredity': Its Influence on the Early Development of Human Genetics." *History of Science* 10 (1971): 1–27.

– "The 'Law of Ancestral Heredity' and the Mendelian-Ancestrian Controversy in England, 1889–1906." *Journal of Medical Genetics* 8 (1971): 1–36.

Gasca, Ann Millán. "The Biology of Numbers: The Correspondence of Vito Volterra on Mathematical Biology." In *The Biology of Numbers: The Correspondence of Vito Volterra on Mathematical Biology*, edited by G. Israel and Ann Millán Gasca, 1–54. Science Networks. Historical Studies 26. Berlin: Birkauser Verlag, 2002.

Gillham, N.W. "Evolution by Jumps: Francis Galton and William Bateson and the Mechanism of Evolutionary Change." *Genetics* 159 (2001): 1383–92.

Gliboff, S. "Gregor Mendel and the Laws of Evolution." *History of Science* 37 (1999): 217–35.

Grasseni, C. "Designer Cows: The Practice of Cattle Breeding between Skill and Standardization." *Society and Animals* 13 (2005): 33–49.

– "Managing Cows: An Ethnography of Breeding Practices and Uses of Reproductive Technology in Contemporary Dairy Farming in Lombardy (Italy)." *Studies in History and Philosophy of Biological and Biomedical Sciences* 38 (2007): 488–510.

– "Skilled Vision: An Apprenticeship in Breeding Aesthetics." *Social Anthropology* 12 (2004): 41–55.

Grey, J. "History of Mathematics and History of Science Reunited?" *Isis* 102 (2011): 511–17.

Gurkiewicz, M., et al. "Too Much Quantification Hinders Creativity." *Science* 324 (2009): 1515.

Hacking, I. "Introductory Essay." In *The Structure of Scientific Revolutions*, 4th edition. Chicago: University of Chicago Press, 2012.

Hartmann, W. "From Mendel to Multi-National in Poultry Breeding." *World's Poultry Science* 45 (1989): 5–26.

Harwood, J. "Introduction to the Special Issue of Biology and Agriculture." *Journal of the History of Biology* 39 (2006): 237–9.

– "On the Genesis of Technoscience: A Case Study of German Agricultural Education." *Perspectives on Science* 13 (2005): 329–51.

Heleski, C.R., and J. Adroaldo. "Animal Science Student Attitudes to Farm Animal Welfare." *Anthrozoos* 19 (2006): 3–16.

Henlein, P. "Cattle Driving from the Ohio Country, 1800–1850." *Agricultural History* 28 (1954): 83–94.

Hill, W.G. "Applications of Population Genetics to Animal Breeding, from Wright and Lush to Genomic Prediction." *Genetics* 196 (2014): http://www.genetics.org/content/196/1/1.

– "Understanding and Using Quantitative Genetic Variation." *Philosophical Transactions of the Royal Society B: Biological Sciences* 365 (2010): 73–85.

Hill, W.G., and M. Kirkpatrick. "What Animal Breeding Has Taught Us about Evolution." *Annual Review of Ecology, Evolution, and Systematics* 41 (2010): 1–19.

Horowitz, R. "Making the Chicken of Tomorrow: Reworking Poultry as Commodities and as Creatures, 1945–1990." In *Industrializing Organisms: Introducing Evolutionary History*, edited by S.R. Schrepfer and P. Scranton. London: Routledge, 2004.

Howell, P. "The Dog Fancy at War: Breeds, Breeding, and Britishness, 1914–1918." *Society and Animals* 21 (2013): 546–67.

Hustak, C. "Got Milk? Dirty Cows, Unfit Mothers, and Infant Mortality, 1880–1940." In *Animal Metropolis: Histories of Human-Animal Relations in Urban Canada*, edited by J. Dean, D. Ingram, and C. Sethna, 189–218. Calgary: University of Calgary Press, 2017.

Kevles, D.J. "The Advent of Animal Patents: Innovation and Controversy in the Engineering and Ownership of Life." In *Intellectual Property Rights in Animal Breeding and Genetics*, edited by M. Rothschild and S. Newman. New York: CABI Publishing, 2002.

– "Patents, Protections, and Privileges." *Isis* 98 (2007): 323–31.

– "Protections, Privileges, and Patents: Intellectual Property in Animals and Plants since the Late Eighteenth Century." In *Con/Texts of Invention*, edited by M. Biagioli, P. Jaszi, and M. Woodmansee. Chicago: University of Chicago Press, 2008.

Johnson, K. "Iowa Dairying at the Turn of the Century: The New Agriculture and Progressivism." *Agricultural History* 45 (1971): 95–110.

Johnson, L.P.V. "Dr. W.J. Spillman's Discoveries in Genetics: An Evaluation of His Pre-Mendelian Experiments with Wheat." *Journal of Heredity* 39 (1948): 247–54.

Jull, A. "Inbreeding and Crossbreeding in Poultry." *Journal of Heredity* 24 (1933): 93–101.

Kimmelman, B. "The American Breeders' Association: Genetics and Eugenics in an Agricultural Context, 1903–1913." *Social Studies of Science* 13 (1983): 163–204.

– "Mr. Blakeslee Builds His Dream House: Agricultural Institutions, Genetics, and Careers 1900–1945." *Journal of the History of Biology* 39 (2006): 241–80.

Kingsland, S.E. "The Battling Botanist: Daniel Trembly MacDougal, Mutation Theory, and the Rise of Experimental Evolutionary Biology in America, 1900–1912." *Isis* 82 (1991): 479–509.

– "Mathematical Figments, Biological Facts: Population Ecology in the Thirties." *Journal of the History of Biology* 19 (1986): 235–56.

Lange, C. "The Making and Remaking of the Arabian Horse – from the Arab Bedouin Horse to the Modern Straight Egyptian." In *Horse Breeds and Human Society: Purity, Identity and the Making of the Modern Horse*, edited by K. Guest and M. Mattfeld, 234–51. London: Routledge Press, 2020.

– "Purity, Nobility, Beauty and Performance: Past and Present Construction of Meaning for the Arabian Horse." In *The Meaning of Horses: Biosocial Encounters*, edited by D.L. Davis and A. Maustad, 39–53. London: Routledge Press, 2016.

Loew, F.M. "Animal Agriculture." In *The Genetic Revolution: Scientific Prospects and Public Perceptions*, edited by B.D. Davis. Baltimore: Johns Hopkins University Press, 1991.

Lush, J. "Genetics and Animal Breeding." In *Genetics in the 20th Century*, edited by L.C. Dunn, 493–525. New York: Macmillan Company, 1951.

Mackay, T.F.C. "Alan Robertson (1920–1989)." *Genetics* 125 (1990): 1–7.

Marie, J. "For Science, Love and Money: The Social Worlds of Poultry and Rabbit Breeding in Britain, 1900–1940." *Social Studies of Science* 38 (2008): 919–36.

Matz, B. "Crossing, Grading, and Keeping Pure: Animal Breeding and Exchange around 1860." *Endeavour* 35 (2011): 7–15.

Mayr, E. "The Nature of the Darwinian Revolution." *Science* 176 (June 1972): 981–9.

– "The Science-Technology Relationship as a Historiographic Problem." *Technology and Culture* 17 (1976): 663–73.

McCormick, V. "Butter and Egg Business: Implications from the Records of a Nineteenth Century Farm Wife." *Ohio History* 100 (1991): 329–35.

McGrew, T.F. "American Breeds of Poultry." In US Department of Agriculture, Bureau of Animal Industry, *Report* (1901): 513–65.

Mendelsohn, J.A. "'Like All That Lives': Biology, Medicine and Bacteria in the Age of Pasteur and Koch." *History and Philosophy of the Life Sciences* 24 (2002): 3–36.

Millais, E. *The Theory and Practice of Rational Breeding*. London: *The Fancier's Gazette*, 1889.

Moore-Colyer, R.F. "Aspects of Horse Breeding and the Supply of Horses in Victorian Britain." *Agriculture History Review* 43 (1995): 47–60.

Müller-Wille, S., and V. Orel. "From Linnaean Species to Mendelian Factors: Elements of Hybridism, 1751–1870." *Annals of Science* 64 (2007): 171–215.

Nash, R. "A Perfect Nicking Pattern." *Humanimalia* 10 (2018): 27–43.

Olby, R. "Mendel No Mendelist?" *History of Science* 12 (1979): 53–72.

Ollivier, L. "Jay Lush: Reflections on the Past." *Lohmann Information* 43 (2008): 3–12.

Orel, V. "Cloning, Inbreeding, and History." *Quarterly Review of Biology* 72 (1997): 437–40.

– "Commemoration of the N.I. Vavilov Centennial at Brno." *Folia Mendelianna* 23 (1988): 37–50.

– "Selection Practice and Theory of Heredity in Moravia before Mendel." *Folia Mendelianna* 12 (1977): 179–99.

– "The Spectre of Inbreeding in the Early Investigation of Heredity." *History and Philosophy of the Life Sciences* 19 (1997): 315–30.

Orel, V., and R.J. Wood. "Early Development in Artificial Selection as a Background to Mendel's Research." *History and Philosophy of the Life Sciences* 3 (1981): 145–70.

– "Scientific Animal Breeding in Moravia before and after the Discovery of Mendel's Theory." *Quarterly Review of Biology* 75 (2000): 149–57.

Orland, B. "Turbo-Cows: Producing a Competitive Animal in the Nineteenth and Early Twentieth Centuries." In *Industrializing Organisms: Introducing Evolutionary History*, edited by S.R. Schrepfer and P. Scranton. London: Routledge, 2004.

Palladino, P. "Between Craft and Science: Plant Breeding, Mendelian Genetics, and British Universities, 1900–1920." *Technology and Culture* 34 (1993): 300–23.

Paul, D.B., and B. Kimmelman. "Mendel in America: Theory and Practice, 1900–1919." In *The American Development of Biology*, edited by R. Rainger, K. Benson, and J. Maienschein. Philadelphia: University of Pennsylvania Press, 1988.

Pauly, P.J. "The Appearance of Academic Biology in Late Nineteenth-Century America." *Journal of the History of Biology* 17 (1984): 369–97.

Pawson, H.C. "Some Agricultural History Salvaged." *Agricultural History Review* 7 (1959): 6–13.

Pemberton, N., and J.-M. Strange. "Dogs and Modernity: Dogs in History and Culture." *European Review of History* 22 (2015): 705–8.

Pemberton, N., and M. Worboys. "The Invention of the Basset Hound: Breed. Blood and the Late Victorian Dog Fancy, 1865–1900." *European Review of History* 22 (2015): 726–40.

Perry, P.J. "The Shorthorn Comes of Age, 1822–1843." *Agricultural History* 56 (1982): 560–6.

Plumb, C.B. "Felix Renick, Pioneer." *Ohio Archaeological and Historical Publications* 38 (1924): 3–66.

Pollott, G.E. "Bioinformatical Genetics – Opening the Black Box of Quantitative Genetics." *Proceedings of the World Congress on Genetics Applied to Livestock Production*, 2006 (23.21).

Preston, R. "The Genome Warrior." *New Yorker*, 12 June 2000, 66–83.

Punnett, R.C. "Early Days of Genetics." *Heredity* 4 (1950): 1–10.

Quinn, M.S. "Corpulent Cows and Milk Machines: Nature, Art and the Ideal Type." *Society and Animals* 1 (1993): 145–57.

Reeve, E. Book review of *Proceedings of the Second International Conference on Quantitative Genetics* by B.S. Weir et al. *Genetical Research* 53 (1989): 239–40.

Rheinberger, H.-J., and P. McLaughlin. "Darwin's Experimental Natural History." *Journal of the History of Biology* 17 (1984): 345–68.

Richards, R.A. "Darwin and the Inefficacy of Artificial Selection." *Studies in History and Philosophy of Science* 28 (1997): 75–97.

Ritvo, H. "Possessing Mother Nature: Genetic Capital in Eighteenth-Century Britain." In *Early Modern Conceptions of Capital*, edited by J. Brewer and S. Staves, 413–26. London: Routledge, 1995.

– "Pride and Pedigree: The Evolution of the Victorian Dog Fancy." *Victorian Studies* 29 (1986): 227–53.

Roll-Hansen, N. "Theory and Practice: The Impact of Mendelism on Agriculture." *C.R. Acad. Sci. Paris, Sciences de la Vie/Life Sciences* 323 (2000): 1107–16.

Rowe, D.J. "The Culleys, Northumberland Farmers 1767–1813." *Agricultural History Review* 19 (1971): 156–74.

Ruse, M. "Charles Darwin and Artificial Selection." *Journal of the History of Ideas* 36 (1975): 339–50.

Ryder, M.L. "The History of Sheep Breeds in Britain." *Agricultural History Review* 12 (1964): part 1: 1–12, part 2: 79–97.

Sapp, Jan. "The Nine Lives of Gregor Mendel." In *Experimental Inquiries: Historical, Philosophical and Social Studies of Experimentation in Science*, edited by H.E. Le Grand, 137–66. Dordrecht: Kluwer Academic Publishers, 1990.

– "The Struggle for Authority in the Field of Heredity, 1900–1932: New Perspectives on the Rise of Genetics." *Journal of the History of Biology* 16 (1983): 311–42.

Secord, J.A. "Nature's Fancy: Charles Darwin and the Breeding of Pigeons." *Isis* 72 (1981): 163–86.

Shrader, H.L. "The Chicken-of-Tomorrow Program: Its Influence on 'Meat-Type' Poultry Production." *Poultry Science* 31 (1952): 3–10.

Skinner, J.L. "150 Years of the Poultry Industry." *World's Poultry Science Journal* 30–1 (1974–5): 27–31.

Sloan, P.R. "Essay Review: Ernst Mayr on the History of Biology." *Journal of the History of Biology* 18 (1985): 145–53.

Stamhuis, I.H., et al. "Hugo de Vries on Heredity, 1889–1903: Statistics, Mendelian Laws, Pangenes, Mutations." *Isis* 90 (1999): 238–67.

Sterrett, S.G. "Darwin's Analogy between Artificial and Natural Selection: How Does It Go?" *Studies in History and Philosophy of Biological and Biomedical Sciences* 33 (2002): 151–68.

Taylor, D. "The English Dairy Industry, 1860–1930." *Economic History Review*, series 2, 29 (1976): 585–601.

– "London's Milk Supply, 1850–1900: A Reinterpretation." *Agricultural History* 45 (1971): 33–8.

Theunissen, L.T.G. "Breeding for Nobility or Production? Cultures of Dairy Cattle Breeding in the Netherlands, 1945–1995." *Isis* 103 (2012): 278–309.

– "Breeding without Mendelism: Theory and Practice of Dairy Cattle Breeding in the Netherlands, 1900–1950." *Journal of the History of Biology* 41 (2008): 637–76.

– "Closing the Door on Hugo de Vries' Mendelism." *Annals of Science* 51 (1994): 225–48.

– "Darwin and His Pigeons: The Analogy between Artificial and Natural Selection Revisited." *Journal of the History of Biology* 45 (2012): 179–212.

– "Knowledge Is Power: Hugo de Vries on Science, Heredity and Social Progress." *British Journal for the History of Science* 27 (1994): 291–331.

– "Practical Animal Breeding as the Key to an Integrated View of Genetics, Eugenics and Evolutionary Theory: Arend L. Hagedoorn (1885–1953)." *Studies in History and Philosophy of Science Part C: Studies in History and Philosophy of Biological and Biomedical Sciences* 46 (2014): 55–64.

– "The Transformation of the Dutch Farm Horse into a Riding Horse: Livestock Breeding, Science, and Modernization, 1960s–1980s." *Agricultural History* 92 (2018): 24–53.

Thompson, F.M.L. "Nineteenth-Century Horse Sense." *Economic History Review*, series 2, 19 (1976): 60–81.

Thurtle, P. "Harnessing Heredity in Gilded Age America: Middle Class Mores and Industrial Breeding in a Cultural Context." *Journal of the History of Biology* 35 (2002): 43–78.

van der Werf, J. "Animal Breeding and the Black Box of Biology." *Journal of Animal Breeding and Genetics* 124 (2007): 101.

Voth, K. "From Big to Small to Big to Small: Part 2 of a Pictorial History of Cattle Changes over the Years." *On Pasture*, 11 July 2016. Based on the research of Harlan Ritchie of Michigan State University on the history of beef cattle styles. Page 1–2. http://onpasture.com/2016/07/11/from-big-to-small-to-big-to-small-part-2-of-a-pictorial-history-of-cattle-changes-over-the-years. Accessed 13 July 2016.

– "From Big to Small to Big to Small: Part 3 of a Pictorial History of Cattle Changes over the Years." *On Pasture*, 18 July 2016. Based on the research of Harlan Ritchie of Michigan State University on the history of beef cattle styles. Page 10–11. http://onpasture.com/2016/07/11/from-big-to-small-to-big-to-small-part-3-of-a-pictoral-history-of-cattle-changes-over-the-years. Accessed 18 July 2016.

Walton, J. "The Diffusion of Improved Shorthorn Cattle in Britain during the Eighteenth and Nineteenth Centuries." *Transactions of the Institute of British Geographers* ns 9 (1984): 22–36.
– "Pedigree and the National Cattle Herd circa 1750–1950." *Agricultural History Review* 34 (1986): 149–70.
Warren, D.C. "A Half Century of Advances in the Genetics and Breeding Improvement of Poultry." *Poultry Science* 37 (1958): 3–20.
Weir, B.S. "Quantitative Genetics in 1987." *Genetics* 117 (1987): 601–2.
Weller, J.I. "Introduction to QTL Detection and Marker-Assisted Selection." In *Biotechnology's Role in the Genetic Improvement of Farm Animals*, edited by R.H. Miller et al., 259–61. Beltsville Symposia in Agricultural Research, American Society of Animal Science, 1996.
Whetham, E. "The Trade in Pedigree Livestock, 1850–1910." *Agricultural History Review* 27 (1979): 47–50.
White, K. "Victorian and Edwardian Dogs." *Veterinary History* ns 7 (1992): 72–8.
Wieland, T. "Scientific Theory and Agricultural Practice: Plant Breeding in Germany from the Late 19th to the Early 20th Century." *Journal of the History of Biology* 39 (2006): 309–43.
Wilmot, S. "Between the Farm and the Clinic: Agricultural and Reproductive Technology in the Twentieth Century." *Studies in History and Philosophy of Biological and Biomedical Sciences* 38 (2007): 303–15.
– "From Public Service to Artificial Insemination: Animal Breeding Science, 1890–1951." Full Research Report, ESRC End of Award Report, Reference No. Res-000-23-0390, pages 14–22. 2007.
– "From 'Public Service' to Artificial Insemination: Animal Breeding Science and Reproductive Research in Early 20th Century Britain." *Studies in History and Philosophy of Biological and Biomedical Sciences* 38 (2007): 411–41.
Wood, R.J. "Robert Bakewell (1725–1795): Pioneer Animal Breeder and His Influence on Charles Darwin." *Folia Mendelianna* 8 (1973): 231–42.
Wood, R.J., and V. Orel. "Scientific Breeding in Central Europe during the Early Nineteenth Century: Background to Mendel's Later Work." *Journal of the History of Biology* 38 (2005): 239–72.
Worboys, M. "Inventing Dog Breeds: Jack Russell Terriers." *Humanimalia* 10 (2018): 44–73.
Wright, S. "The Genetic Theory of Natural Selection." *Journal of Heredity* 21 (1930): 349–56.
– "Mendelian Analysis of the Pure Bred Breeds of Livestock, Part 1: The Measurement of Inbreeding and Relationship." *Journal of Heredity* 14 (1923): 339–48.
– "Mendelian Analysis of the Pure Bred Breeds of Livestock, Part 2: The Duchess Family of Shorthorns As Bred by Thomas Bates." *Journal of Heredity* 14 (1923): 405–22.

– "The Relation of Livestock Breeding to Theories of Evolution." *Journal of Animal Science* 46 (1978): 1192–1200.

Wykes, D. "Robert Bakewell (1725–1795) of Dishley: Farmer and Livestock Improver." *Agricultural History Review* 52 (2004): 38–55.

Yi, Doogab. "Who Owns What? Private Ownership and the Public Interest in Recombinant DNA Technology in the 1970s." *Isis* 102 (2011): 446–74.

Index